JAKE'S PRAYER

I pray for wisdom, for harmony,
for concordance and unity with
all those I come in contact with.
I pray that God's presence will
surround and encompass all that is
being around me and ask the Lord
to allow me to step back and
recognize his influence over
people and places and
things in my life.

Be with me Lord. Open my life
to new directions and possibilities

Help me to understand why
there is a moth on my left sleeve.

For all those I have loved, continue
to love, will always love,
and those I have yet to love
because in the end there is only love

2/23/09

This handwritten prayer was found among Jake's belongings after his death.

THE

Book OF

Whispers

A Father and Son's Battle with Bipolar Disorder

THE STORY OF MICKEY AND JAKE McCLAIN DRIVER

AS TOLD TO BEVERLY FREEMAN

The events in this account of Jake's life are factual, however, names of certain
individuals and institutions have been changed or not disclosed.

All profits from *The Book of Whispers* benefit the National Alliance on Mental Illness
Greater Houston, www.namigreaterhouston.org.

Printed in the United States of America

May 2016

Designed by Artisan Field, Inc. Houston, Texas
www.artisanfield.com

To my son Jake, whom I love more than anything,
and who taught me to open my heart bigger than I could
have ever imagined. Through his struggles, I learned the difference
between what is important in life and what is not. I am so proud of
him and what he accomplished in the face of so many challenges.
He taught me the true meaning of unconditional love.

And to my wife, best friend, love of my life and soulmate, Debbie.
Through the worst of everything, she has been my strength and
encouragement, making sure I keep all matters of life and death
in perspective. She, too, knows the pain and grief of losing a child.
And to all people everywhere who have been, and continue to be,
touched by mental illness. You are not alone.

INDEX

INTRODUCTION

The Book of Whispers is the story of a young man's courageous battle with bipolar disorder.

It was a battle he lost.

But not without a fight.

Like so many of the nearly ten million Americans suffering from this insidious disease, Jake McClain Driver was a talented, passionate, brilliant young man with a tortured mind. His creativity and wit were astonishing. He was a gifted writer and played amazing guitar. He wrote songs and poetry, painted, drew and made pieces of art. He had a great sense of humor, an innate ability to connect with others, and as a result, he loved and was loved.

Jake also had an illness. One moment he was sweet, loving and engaging. In the next, he was agitated, erratic and disruptive. He worked hard to overcome his problems. He went to numerous doctors who prescribed a myriad of treatment plans involving medications and therapy. He was hospitalized multiple times. He was shot by a police officer. He served time in jail. Finally, at age 26, he took his own life.

In spite of his debilitating illness, Jake continued to create. Among his creative efforts were a series of poems that he compiled into a book he called *The Book of Whispers*. No one knows why he gave his book of poetry that name, however, those of us who were close to Jake believe that his verses may have been whispers to him that helped silence or quiet the chaos in his head that he experienced with his disease.

Through his poetry, Jake weaves his own personal experience as he battles demons and pain that might seem unfathomable to others. Some of the verses are whimsical and downright funny. Others are thought provoking. A few are sad. They are presented here as he wrote them, with all lower case letters and with titles underlined.

When we began to consider publishing Jake's book, the goal was simply to share his poetry with others. As the project progressed, we came to understand that the poetry is even more meaningful when read within the context of Jake's all-too-short life. Unfortunately, Jake is not able to tell his story himself, so I am telling it for him from my perspective as his father and a caregiver of a child with mental illness.

Jake had an illness that killed him. It is an illness that is not understood or accepted. Yet, for those who must live with it, it is as real as cancer or heart disease. And just like other physical illnesses, it is often fatal.

Today, bipolar disorder has become almost trendy thanks to the public struggles of many famous creative high achievers who are artists, writers and actors. But in spite of increased public awareness, mental illness continues to be a source of misinformation and embarrassment. For those who are ill and their loved ones, there is no glamour – only pain, broken dreams, and often discrimination.

According to the National Alliance on Mental Illness (NAMI), 2.6 percent of Americans, or more than 10 million people living in the United States, suffer from bipolar disorder. Around the globe, it is estimated that 250 million people potentially have the disease. Yet, most people have only the vaguest knowledge of it.

It is not a new problem. Throughout history, individuals who suffered from this illness were called "mad" or were said to be suffering from "melancholia." In more modern times, terms such as manic-depressive disorder have been used.

Whatever you call it, bipolar disorder is a serious brain disorder that causes severe mood swings that range from deep depression to manic highs. These mood swings cause dramatic changes in energy and activity levels that can seriously impair an individual's judgment and their ability to function.

Bipolar disorder often plays a role in violence and serious crimes. Individuals suffering from the disease are at significantly greater risk for developing substance abuse problems and attention-deficit disorder. They may also experience psychotic episodes such as hallucinations or delusions.

This disorder is also one of the leading causes of suicide. About 15 percent of those who are diagnosed with bipolar disorder will kill themselves and many of those who do so will die while abusing drugs or alcohol.

The median age for diagnosis is around 25, but most who develop the disease exhibit symptoms much younger. Many struggle for years through the medical and mental health systems before receiving an accurate diagnosis. Even once a diagnosis is received, the road ahead is rough. This is a long-term illness and finding effective medications and therapies is an ongoing effort.

A parent's journey with a child who is suffering from bipolar disorder is a difficult one fraught with enough challenges to fill an entire library. They are overwhelmed by problems and consumed with guilt. They give up considerable time, energy and financial resources, often with very little to show for it.

It is also a journey filled with moments of great joy and love.

By publishing *The Book of Whispers,* we remember the joy and love we shared with Jake and the unique gifts he shared with us. He touched many lives and will be remembered always by those who knew him as an inspiration for his courage and strength in dealing with so many disappointments and adversities in his life.

Most of all, we hope that Jake's story may make a difference to others. If even one person who is fighting to survive the ravages of mental illness – their own or that of a loved one – is helped by hearing about Jake's journey or by reading his poetry, the effort to publish it will have been worth it.

CHAPTER 1

EVERYTHING SEEMS POSSIBLE

"i can take as much credit for my creations
as my parents can for my flesh and blood"

FROM JAKE'S POEM "A TRUE POET SPEAKS"

The best day of your life is the day your child is born. Anything – and everything – seems possible.

You fall in love the moment you hold him in your arms for the first time. You are brimming with joy. Your thoughts race ahead to the wondrous future that this tiny being will experience. He can be anything he wants to be. He can do anything he wants to do. And you will be there to applaud his success and to help him navigate the bumps along the way.

It was that way the day Jake McClain Driver was born.

Jake came into the world on a beautiful, crystal-clear, blue-sky Saturday morning, February 26, 1983, at Northside Hospital in Atlanta, Georgia. His "due date" wasn't for another two weeks, but Jake decided that this would be his day.

He was absolutely perfect in every way. He had his mom's red curly hair and a great set of lungs. We both fell in love with him at once. His mother, Anne, and I couldn't wait to take him home and start our new life as a family.

We named him Jake because we liked the name and we wanted something simple and short. Unfortunately, we allowed ourselves to be influenced by friends who made fun of the name. They said it sounded too countrified. So we named him Jared instead. But we always called him Jake, and eventually, we changed the name on his birth certificate from Jared to Jake.

I was thrilled to have a son. He was great fun to play with. I told everyone that he was the best toy I ever had – and I didn't have to put batteries in him!

Anne and I were enthralled by his efforts to walk and talk. He did everything exactly as he was supposed to. He walked on time and talked

1

on time. My heart melted when his first word was "da da" and his vocabulary grew quickly with each passing day. He was never shy. He could talk to anybody and was exceedingly good company.

He was a born performer with a vivid imagination. He rode the western range on his rocking horse, describing his adventures as a cowboy to the world at large. After an evening at the circus, he would entertain us with imitations of the announcer, serving as ringmaster of his own imaginary circus.

His interest in reading began in his mother's womb. I read to Anne's growing tummy every night while she was pregnant, and when he was young, our reading time was a special part of our day. I read dozens of Golden Books aloud to him in the evenings until he learned to read them for himself. As he got older, we read the newspapers together, and he continued his interest in news and current events for the rest of his life.

When Jake was just a few months old, I was transferred from Atlanta to Nashville where I worked as a lobbyist for Gulf Oil Corporation. Two years later, Gulf was bought by Chevron and I was offered a job in Chevron's Public Affairs office in San Francisco. We settled into our new home in Walnut Creek in the East Bay, and Jake blossomed into a normal, active little boy.

As parents of an only child, we were naturally very protective and monitored his progress carefully. We watched what he ate and made sure that he was exposed to as many educational and cultural experiences as possible.

Our protectiveness extended to his toys. Jake was not allowed to play with toys that involved any form of violence; however, one day when he was about three years old, a friend came over with his arsenal of toy guns. They were playing in the backyard playhouse, and Jake kept getting shot because he didn't have a toy gun to defend himself. Anne and I weighed the influence of playing with toy guns against our desire for him to be normal and to fit in with other children. In the end, we decided it was perfectly normal for little boys to play soldier. The next day, I took him to Toys R Us and bought him toy guns and a toy sword. From that point on, Jake was able to defend himself on the playground.

Jake exhibited an interest in music when he was very young. He had fun dressing up like Michael Jackson with hat, glove, jacket and microphone and singing "Thriller." I had grown up in a home that was filled with people making music. In the 1940s, my dad had his own country band, Jimmie Driver and the Tennessee Playboys, which toured the South and played on the Grand Ole Opry. During my childhood, we had a family band made up of my dad, mom, my five brothers and myself. I wanted to share this heritage with Jake, so when he was five years old, I bought him a ukulele. He took to it at once. I taught him a few chords, and he learned to play several simple songs.

His first public performance came on July 4, 1988, while we were attending the Fiddlers' Jamboree and Crafts Festival in my hometown of Smithville, Tennessee. This annual event features two days of food and handmade crafts, and the main attraction is a bluegrass music competition on a big stage in the public square in the middle of town.

We were listening to some of the performers when Jake suddenly tugged on my hand. "I want to play my song!" he told me. He had recently learned a country song released by Alabama called *Song of the South* and he loved to sing it. I was a little dubious, but I asked the organizers if he could sing and they said okay. I borrowed my dad's guitar, got Jake's ukulele and we walked onto the stage. The microphone was placed down at Jake's level and he sang with gusto:

> Song, song of the South,
> Sweet potato pie and I shut my mouth
> Gone, gone with the wind
> There ain't nobody looking back again

He bowed to great applause as we finished the last chorus. Jake was delighted with his debut, and I was impressed with his confidence on the stage.

Back home in California, it was time for Jake to start school. Because Jake's birthday was in late February, we had to make a decision about whether he would start kindergarten or pre-kindergarten. Instead of placing him in kindergarten where he would be among the youngest in his class, we decided on the option to start him one school year later so that he would be among the oldest in his grade.

He entered pre-kindergarten at Seven Hills, a private school in Walnut Creek. The school had a strong artistic program and fit perfectly with Jake's creative interests. He increased his reading and writing abilities quickly and made lots of new friends.

There were absolutely no issues; no warning signs. He was a smart, energetic, precocious little boy. We never thought that anything would change.

CHAPTER 2

IF I KNEW THEN WHAT I KNOW NOW...

"the universe is all voices
yet it cannot speak for itself
it speaks through you
you are the universe"

FROM JAKE'S POEM "ONE"

It is hard to put your finger on the time when things start to go wrong in a marriage, but at some point during the time that we lived in California, Anne and I began having serious marital problems.

Achieving success in large companies like Chevron requires employees to relocate, and by the time Jake started pre-school, we had been transferred from Houston to Atlanta, from Atlanta to Nashville, and from Nashville to San Francisco. The toll of moving and corporate life was beginning to weigh heavily on Anne, and she was changing how she viewed the world.

Anne and I grew up in DeKalb County in the rolling green hills of Middle Tennessee. I lived on a farm with my parents and five brothers near the small town of Smithville, population 4,000. Our family grew tobacco, peanuts and other crops and raised beef and dairy cattle. Growing up, I milked cows and did chores around the farm. For fun, we hunted rabbits and squirrels, and on weekends, we played guitars, fiddles and mandolins. My maternal grandparents and a couple of aunts and uncles lived nearby. We became city folks when we moved to Smithville about the time I started high school.

Anne and I met at the local swimming pool in Smithville and went on a couple of dates with friends. We began dating seriously when she entered the University of Tennessee at Knoxville to study fashion merchandising just a few months before I finished my degree in journalism and mass communications. After graduation, I returned to Smithville to work for the U.S. Government's Model Cities program, but we continued to date throughout her college years.

Anne was very smart and pretty, with long strawberry blonde hair. In high school, she was a cheerleader and salutatorian of her senior class. In college, she had an almost perfect grade point average. She was inducted into the Phi Beta Kappa National Honor Society and was a leader in her Pi Beta Phi sorority.

After she graduated, I resigned my job with the Model Cities program. On December 31, 1972, we loaded the car and headed to Houston where Anne had been hired to work in fashion merchandising management at Sakowitz, an upscale Houston department store. We arrived on New Year's Day 1973 and were excited about starting out together in a new city on the first day of a new year. Houston was booming in the early 1970s, and I quickly found a job as the editor of the employee publications at Transcontinental Gas Pipe Line Corporation. Anne settled into her new job and her career was going well.

The decision to get married was very spontaneous. We had been living together somewhat secretly since moving to Houston, and now, her mother was coming to visit. Just prior to her arrival, Anne said, "Why don't we get married while my mother is here?"

We were married at noon on Wednesday, May 9, 1973, in a small ceremony at St. Martin's Episcopal Church on Sage Road. Anne's mother served as matron of honor and a female friend from work was my "best man." Our honeymoon consisted of driving to Galveston that evening for a romantic dinner at the Flagship Hotel overlooking the Gulf of Mexico. The next morning, we went back to work.

We settled comfortably into domestic life and both did well in our careers. I continued to work in Houston's burgeoning energy industry, eventually joining Shell Oil's public affairs staff and then moving to the public affairs department at Gulf Oil in 1976. After a few years in the Houston office, Gulf transferred us to Atlanta.

While in Houston, Anne worked at Sakowitz and later at Joske's, two of the city's finer department stores. Then, she made a career change to teach retailing in high school as part of the Distributive Education Clubs of America (DECA). Later, when we moved to Atlanta, she taught fashion merchandising at the Art Institute of Atlanta.

It was during our time in Atlanta that Anne first became interested in New Age ideologies. In the beginning, she just dabbled in it, but when Gulf transferred us from Atlanta to Nashville a few years later, her interest deepened. By the time we were transferred to California in 1985, she was deep into New Age philosophies and beliefs.

In California, Anne became a representative for Beauty Control Cosmetics and was offered a car for her outstanding sales record. At the same time, she explored past lives, channeled spirits and became increasingly involved in hands-on healing. She truly believed that she had the gift of placing her hands on a person and channeling healing powers into their cancer or other ailment. She took classes and attended seminars on clairvoyance, healing abilities, reiki, crystal therapy and chakra balancing just to name a few.

This was not who Anne was when we married. This was something new that I was finding challenging to accept on an everyday basis. Many people have such beliefs, but I did not, and not sharing the same beliefs caused a strain in our relationship. We began to argue about it, especially when she tried to involve Jake. He was at a very impressionable age, and I was concerned about his mother telling him that he had just been reborn or that she had the gift of healing.

Like many married couples, we also argued about money. I was concerned about her spending habits, and she thought I was stingy. It tore at the fabric of our marriage, and over time, our relationship began to disintegrate.

Like so many couples struggling with marital issues, we put on a good front when it came to Jake and our family and friends. We loved Jake and enjoyed being parents, taking him camping several times at Lake Tahoe, to Webelo Scout meetings, soccer games, Disneyland, the La Brea Tar Pits and other fun places all over California.

In early 1990, I was delighted to learn that we were being transferred back to Houston. We had loved living in the city in the 1970s, and I thought it would help to get Anne away from the epicenter of New Age influences in the San Francisco Bay Area.

While we lived in California, Anne's mother was a frequent visitor, and now, she came to stay with Jake while Anne and I flew to Houston to search for a house. We found a beautiful property in the Memorial area on Houston's west side where we decided to build a new custom home. We signed the paperwork and went back to California to prepare for what I swore would be our final move. We kissed her mother goodbye and commenced packing.

It was late Sunday afternoon, April 1 – the day before the moving trucks were coming – when we got a call from the Sheriff's Department in Smithville. Anne's mother had been found at her home, dead from a self-inflicted gunshot wound.

Anne's sister in Nashville had not heard from her mom for several days and became concerned. When she couldn't get in touch with her, she asked the Sheriff's Department to check on her. She was 67.

We were stunned. The family was aware that she had suffered from time to time with depression, but the possibility of suicide had not been considered. Not once was there a hint that she was thinking of taking her life.

Anne, Jake and I flew immediately to Tennessee, leaving the moving company to take care of the packing. Jake was very sad at the loss of his "Ninny," but we did not discuss the circumstances of his grandmother's death with him in detail. At seven, he was too young to understand.

It was after the funeral, in a conversation with some members of the family, that I learned for the first time that Anne's grandfather, Jake's great grandfather, had also committed suicide with a gun. I was shocked and upset at the news. No one had ever mentioned this before, and now, no one would talk about it. When I tried to ask questions, Anne's sister said simply, "I think he was depressed. We really don't know very much about it."

At the time, I wasn't especially concerned for Jake's sake. It was only later that I learned that while scientists have not determined exactly what causes bipolar disorder, there is a high probability of a genetic predisposition to the disease. Research has shown that while having a family member who is bipolar does not mean that you will necessarily develop the disease, about 80 to 90 percent of those diagnosed as bipolar have a family history that includes either bipolar disorder or major depression.

If I had known then what I know now, I might have been worried.

Would it have changed things?

I'll never know.

THE THINGS YOU'LL NEVER KNOW

"i see the wind
the wind is beautiful
the wind is like god"

FROM JAKE'S POEM "GOD"

For the survivors of those who have succumbed to mental illness, it's the things you'll never know that are the most troubling.

How did my loved one get this disease?

Was it hereditary?

Did he have it from birth or was there an event that triggered it?

Was it something I did? Or didn't do?

What caused this awful change in my child, spouse, brother or sister?

What could I have done to keep this from happening?

The fact is that most of us will never have the answers to a thousand questions about our loved one and bipolar disorder. Even knowing when it started is not an easy question to answer. For some parents, there is a feeling at an early age that something isn't quite right or a sense that the person is deeply disturbed. But in Jake's case there was nothing to predict what was coming.

When we arrived back in Houston in 1990, Jake had just completed kindergarten in Walnut Creek. We searched for a similar private school in Houston and decided on St. Francis Episcopal Day School. He started first grade there in the fall of 1990. He was smart and scored in the top tier of students in all of his classes and activities. He made new friends and enjoyed the opportunities offered by the school to be creative.

We lived in a great neighborhood with lots of boys and girls his age. They played constantly, skate boarding, climbing trees and playing baseball. He played on a Pee Wee baseball team with boys his age. Not only was he a good player, but it was also a great social outlet for him. He enjoyed the games and parties and hanging out with his friends.

He was also interested in learning to play the guitar. I had taught him a few chords on my guitar and had bought him a small acoustic guitar for practice. Soon he was learning chords and songs on his own. Next came a red, Ibanez electric guitar. With that, Jake started playing riffs and picking out songs. It was evident he had a natural gift for learning and playing music.

I was happy to be back in Houston where I was Chevron's public affairs manager responsible for media, community and government relations. Work was going well. Among my public affairs duties was to represent the company in the community, and I served on the boards of a number of Houston's arts and charitable organizations. Anne and I had a busy social schedule, attending dinners and events on Chevron's behalf.

I also served on several national boards, including the American Hispanic Family of the Year. Each year, First Lady Barbara Bush, who served as honorary chairman of the organization, invited members of the board of directors to a White House reception. Anne, Jake and I were invited to attend this special event held in the Blue Room. We were awed by our historic surroundings and impressed with the warmth of Mrs. Bush, who was a very gracious hostess.

Jake was allowed to accompany us and while he seemed nonplussed by his surroundings, he behaved well. Millie, the Bush's Springer Spaniel, had the run of the place, and before long, she and Jake were great friends. The White House photographer joined me in taking photos of Jake playing with Millie on the floor. It was a very special day for our family.

Unfortunately, our marriage did not fare as well as my career. The marital problems that had begun in Atlanta and continued to fester in Nashville and California followed us to Texas. Over the next three years, we worked with marriage counselors individually, as a couple and as a family, all to no avail. The unhappiness grew as we each solidified our beliefs and values, which the other did not share. On one particularly bad day, Jake used duct tape to make a line down the middle of the house and labeled one half "Mommy's side" and the other half "Daddy's side."

It was during this time that Jake began to complain of stomach pain. There was nothing specific, just "my stomach hurts." It was a mantra that would continue for the rest of his life. Doctor after doctor could find nothing wrong. We took him to gastrointestinal specialists who ran endless tests. No one could find anything wrong, except Anne.

Anne felt that Jake was channeling negative energy, and against my wishes, she took him to a faith healer who prescribed "surgery." During this "procedure," the healer said he would reach inside Jake's body with his hands and pull out the offending object that was causing him pain. Jake was terrified when his mother proposed the idea to him, and I was furious with her for frightening him.

Meanwhile, in August, we enrolled Jake at Briargrove Elementary School. Over the next few months, Anne and I gradually reached the conclusion that our marriage was not going to survive, even though we had both worked long and hard to find solutions to our problems. We no longer shared the same goals, ideals and beliefs that were the cornerstones of our marriage. After weeks of discussing how to proceed, Anne moved out to a nearby apartment and took Jake with her. We decided that I would stay with the house and sell it as soon as possible.

I was devastated. I don't believe in divorce, and I grieved over the failure of our 20-year marriage. Of equal importance, I was sad about a future where I would not be there for Jake every day.

My concern about not being with Jake was relatively short lived. After only two weeks, Anne called and told me to pick up Jake. He was behaving badly and was driving her crazy. I was only too happy to have him come to live with me.

Our divorce progressed through arbitration. I gave Anne about 95 percent of everything she wanted, including alimony (not required in the State of Texas), child support for the periods when Jake lived with her, and 60 percent of my Chevron savings and pension accounts. I assumed all debt and would stay in our new custom-built house until it was sold. I would also pay all of her expenses.

Shortly after the arbitration agreement was completed and before our divorce was final, she moved to a New Age commune near Hot Springs, Arkansas. On January 3, 1994, I appeared in court alone. Anne's lawyer represented her, and a judge signed our divorce papers. Our marriage was over.

Jake turned 11 in February, and he and I settled into a quiet routine. For his birthday, I gave him an acoustical guitar and a flight on a small airplane out of West Houston Airport. I had gotten my private pilot's license in the early 1980s and was always interested in airplanes, so I wanted to share that interest with Jake. I arranged with a pilot instructor at the airport to take Jake on a one-hour training flight around Houston. Jake was excited not only to fly in the Cessna 172, but also to learn about the controls. He was allowed to sit in the pilot's seat and actually maneuver the plane by following the pilot's instructions. I had a special certificate made for him, signed by the pilot, attesting to Jake's flight and training. He also received a pilot's logbook with his first hour of flight training noted.

On our weekends at home together, we went to libraries, plays, concerts, museums, festivals and Houston Rockets basketball games. We cheered the Rockets on at all of their playoff games leading up to the 1995 NBA National Championship. I had grown up in the church, and now, Jake and I attended Sunday services together. While the divorce was heartbreaking, there began to be some semblance of a new beginning that provided hope for a better, and happier, future.

Meanwhile, I was becoming romantically involved with Debbie, a woman I had met at work. We had known each other professionally at Chevron, and over time, we began to date. Although she was almost 11 years younger than me, we had a lot in common – she was a single parent of two boys, pretty and smart, but very practical and down to earth.

Jake found out that we were dating and he was terribly upset. He was very protective of his mom, and sensing that this was a serious relationship, he made it clear that he did not care for Debbie and he opposed our relationship. In the beginning, I made the mistake of not telling Jake when I was going on a date with Debbie, and that deception made things even worse. When Jake would find out that I had been out with her, he would act out, causing me all kinds of grief.

Debbie understood to a point, but it put a strain on our developing relationship. We would break up, then get back together, then break up again. She felt particularly hurt in 1996 when I took Jake on several trips, but did nothing with her. It took several years, but in early 1997 when my 53-year-old brother, Randy, died in a motorcycle accident, I came to my senses. I stopped the "don't tell Jake" nonsense and took Debbie to my brother's funeral in Tennessee. From then on, she was, and has been, the love of my life.

Anne was also moving on with her life. While living at the commune in Arkansas, she met a man who shared her New Age interests, and they became involved. After several months together in Arkansas, they married and moved back to Houston where they lived in an apartment near Jake and me. Of course, Anne wanted Jake to move in with them. Jake had missed his mom during her absence and wanted to be with her, so reluctantly, I agreed.

The next few months were tough on everyone. Jake and Anne's new husband did not get along. The three of them were receiving family counseling and Jake's stomach pain was getting progressively worse.

Conversely, Debbie was rightly concerned by Jake's behavior. While he never actually harmed her, he would make childish threats or react by throwing things. Debbie became particularly upset when he threatened to use his bee-bee gun to shoot her son, Billy. I took the gun away and he never got it back.

At age 11, Jake was smart and articulate and he made good grades. He made lots of friends and was doing well with one exception – the stomach pain kept getting worse.

As the school year drew to a close, he starred in Briargrove's theatrical production "There's No Business Like Show Business." He performed "50 States in Rhyme," singing and dancing all over the stage. The principal told the crowd, "This is a very talented young man. Mark my words, he's going to be a star one day."

At home, Jake loved being in his room, and he often sought refuge there. Looking back, I believe he may have suffered from separation anxiety. At an age when most boys are anxious to have sleepovers – and Jake was invited to many at the homes of friends – he would only sleep at home in his own bed. Several times, I picked him up at midnight from a friend's house so he could come home to his own space.

13

On another occasion, Jake was invited to join a friend and his family on a ski trip. One day into the trip, I got a call from Jake pleading with me to come and get him. He was calling from a payphone somewhere in New Mexico and he desperately wanted to come home. It was only after much talking that I persuaded him to continue with the trip.

It was just one more sign that the approaching storm clouds were growing darker.

THE WARNING SIGNS

"i am jumping constantly and could never
interrupt the action to question the pedestal
from which i sprang."

FROM JAKE'S POEM "THIS MORNING'S HIGH"

By age 11, Jake's behavior was becoming more and more erratic. Sometimes, he was defiant and hostile. He refused to be disciplined or to comply with requests made by adults. He thought his teachers were stupid and that he was smarter than they were. At other times, he could be sweet and loving. My heart would melt when he would wrap his arms around me and say, "I love you, Dad."

His stomach pain was getting progressively worse, and by the time he entered his preteen years, it became so severe that Anne was convinced that he needed to be evaluated by a child psychologist. I was somewhat dubious about taking this step. Like most people, I knew almost nothing about mental illness, and I immediately rushed to judgment when it came to involving psychologists in our problems. If you are seeing a psychologist, I thought, there must be something seriously wrong with your mental health. Maybe you are unstable, dysfunctional or even crazy. I was also aware of the stigma attached to mental illness in this country and that many people have negative attitudes and stereotypes when it comes to those suffering with these problems. I did not want my son to be stuck with that label and to experience the prejudice and discrimination that is directed at the mentally ill just because he went to see a psychologist.

But we were also at our wits end when it came to Jake's stomach problems and his behavior. Years of consulting with gastrointestinal specialists and a myriad of other doctors had yielded no answers. Yet, he complained of stomach pain almost every day. He had become very stubborn and did not want to do much of anything. We had to beg him to come out of his room. Finally, I gave in, and a psychologist at West Oaks Hospital evaluated Jake. The psychologist found nothing seriously wrong with Jake's behavior. He felt that given the divorce and all of the things Jake had experienced over the past few years, what he was doing was a normal reaction. We were stumped.

As the end of school year approached, I decided it was time to take Jake on a trip where we could have some fun and, hopefully, forget about his problems for a while. We decided to go to Alaska to hike in Denali National Park.

In June 1995, we flew to Anchorage where we visited all of the usual tourist spots. Next, we headed toward Talkeetna, a small Alaskan village of about 700 that was the inspiration for the television series, *Northern Exposure*. In Talkeetna, I booked a flightseeing tour around Mount McKinley, North America's highest peak with a summit elevation of more than 20,000 feet. We soared above the gentle foothills and rugged peaks of the Alaska Range before landing on a glacier where we got out to play in the snow and throw snowballs at each other. It was a clear day, and we were just a few miles from the summit of the Great One as the Alaskans call Mt. McKinley. The scenery was breathtaking, and Jake was enjoying every minute of it.

After Mt. McKinley, we headed to Denali where we stayed at the Denali Princess Wilderness Lodge. We had a great time hiking the local trails and around the perimeter of the park. Sitting high on one of the hilltops, we could see for miles. It was wonderful to see Jake having so much fun and I loved every moment spent with him.

Since he was not living with me during this period, I made sure I spent as much time with Jake as possible. We continued our tradition of going to Houston Rockets games, and once again, cheered them on to their second consecutive national championship.

Then, Anne and her husband separated. He moved out, and out of the blue, she called one day to tell me that she was moving back to California to be closer to the New Age culture and was taking Jake with her. I was upset, but after I calmed down, I decided not to try to stop her. Given the history of Jake going back and forth between us, I hoped that he would be back with me sooner rather than later.

Four days later, I took them to the airport and watched Anne and Jake's plane take off for the West Coast. I didn't know when I would see him again and I cried all the way home.

Once he was settled in California, I sent cards and letters. I called often. And I begin to worry. By now, Jake was a pre-teen and puberty was hitting with full force. I found it increasingly difficult to talk with him on the phone and, like most kids of this impressionable age, he was too busy with his new friends and new school to have much time for his old dad. I sensed something was not quite right, but it was extremely difficult to determine the problem from a distance.

Jake loved California. Anne had settled in Tiburon across the Bay from San Francisco and enrolled Jake in the sixth grade at Del Mar Middle School. He quickly made friends and channeled his creativity into writing a movie script he called "Alien Cows." He persuaded several of his friends to play parts in the movie he was going to make.

He also loved it when Robin Williams came by the school to say hello to everyone. Williams had grown up and now lived in the Tiburon area, and he often gave his time to visit area schools and entertain at events for local organizations.

Anne's ex-husband joined them in California, and the old problems began again. However, Jake was older now and his reactions were becoming more intense. He did not like Anne's husband and resented that he was living with them again. Anne told me that he was "acting up" by throwing things, being destructive and refusing to go to school. He would not do anything with them or go with them anywhere. The problems continued to escalate until March 1996 when she admitted him to an adolescent mental health hospital in Mill Valley for an evaluation. He remained there for a week.

During his stay, I happened to be in San Francisco on business and visited Jake at the hospital. He was calm and subdued and told me he was plotting routes to escape the hospital. "The other kids here are crazy," he told me. "I've got to get out of here."

That weekend he did get out. There was no diagnosis of any problem. I took him to Lake Tahoe where we went skiing. We skied all day on Saturday; then, we spent several hours at a great restaurant called Jake's on the Lake overlooking Lake Tahoe. Jake could not have been happier.

Back in Houston, my frustration with the distance from Jake and with the lack of information was continuing to grow. Then, Anne suddenly called. She was fed up with Jake's antics and told me: "If you want Jake, buy him a ticket and get him on a plane as soon as you can." I called her back within the hour with travel arrangements. I met Jake as he got off the plane, and once again, he came to live with me.

It was Spring 1996 and he was happy to be back, but a couple of things upset him. During his absence, I had sold the large house we owned in the Memorial area and moved to an apartment. I had recreated Jake's room from the house with his bunk beds and other favorite things, which he liked, but he was furious when he learned that I had given away his dog. I had agreed to keep the dog with me when Anne and Jake moved to California so he would not have to be given away. I was trying to keep the poor animal for Jake, but it didn't have much of a life. I worked all day, and I had to leave the dog alone in a cage. Just weeks before Anne's call, I had decided that the little dog would be better off with a family and had found him a new home. Jake also missed his friends in California, especially the fun he had in putting his "Alien Cows" film together with them.

The apartment that I had moved to after selling the house was only temporary. I had purchased a new patio home that was under construction in a gated community near the Galleria. Jake needed to finish sixth grade, and he was assigned to Grady Middle School in the Spring Branch Independent School District. He finished the sixth grade there and we settled in for some summer fun.

We took a number of trips together that summer, including one to the McIlhenny Tabasco plant on Louisiana's famed Avery Island. Jake loved Tabasco sauce, often smothering his favorite fried chicken and mashed potatoes with the fiery liquid. We had a great time touring the plant to observe how Tabasco is made and visiting local shops that sold many different types of hot sauces with decorative and funny labels. Jake immediately decided that he needed to start a collection and purchased as many as I would allow.

Jake developed a newfound passion for rock climbing. Rock climbing is a physically and mentally challenging sport that tests the climber's endurance, strength and agility, and he loved it. We traveled to rock climbing facilities all around the Houston area and to an old grain silo in Dallas that had been developed into a climbing adventure. We took a trip to El Paso where

Jake climbed the nearby Hueco tanks, a world famous range of low mountains that is widely regarded as one of the best areas for rock climbing in the world.

While we were in the mountains, we decided that it would be fun to hike some of the beautiful trails that traverse Hueco Tanks State Park. We had been warned about rattlesnakes in the area, so Jake and I agreed upon a signal if we should encounter one on the trail. I told him to jump away from the snake and yell "snake, snake, snake."

On a beautiful morning, we were hiking through this sacred desert sanctuary with its natural rock basins and magnificent scenery when Jake suddenly yelled out, "Snake, snake, snake!" A huge rattlesnake was coiled up on the trail right in front of him.

We scrambled down the trail quickly, leaving the snake behind, but it occurred to me that it would be a good idea if we had walkie-talkies so that we could communicate when we were climbing and hiking. I suggested to Jake that he get his amateur radio (also known as ham radio) license. I was an avid amateur radio operator, and I thought it would not only be helpful in situations like the one we just encountered, but it could also be something fun for us to do together.

Jake thought that was a great idea and started studying for his license right away. We bought books and a computer program for him to study and he passed his test with 100 percent accuracy. In November 1996, at age 13, he received his Technician Class license and was issued the call sign KC5WXA. He immediately got a Yaesu FT-50 handy talkie (hand-held radio) and started talking to other hams on it. Jake enjoyed being on the air and kept logbooks of his contacts with other radio operators.

We had fun working together, building antennas, radios, and various types of electronic equipment kits from Radio Shack and Electronic Parts Outlet. He bought a remote controlled car that he would race up and down the street outside of our house. He configured a remote camera and transmitter kit to fit on the car so he could see where it was going and figured out how to transmit a signal from the camera to the television inside the house. He would look out of the window to see someone coming down the street and run the car directly towards them. People didn't know where the car was coming from. He thought it was really funny to sit inside and watch their reactions.

He also built model rockets and became an active member of the Estes Model Rocket Club. On weekends, we would drive out to the big open fields west of Houston and launch these homemade missiles into the sky. Jake was excited to watch his latest rocket shoot into space and reach the peak of its capability. Then, a parachute would deploy and it would come plummeting back to earth. He gave each rocket a name and painted each one with colorful bands and designs.

During this period, he developed a close friendship with a boy from school named Justin. The two of them shared a special bond and he was the only friend with whom Jake would spend the night. Over the summer, they spent a lot of time together, doing magic tricks, shooting hoops, swimming and generally just hanging out and being boys. Every weekend we would choose a place to go and head out on the next adventure around town, and Justin often accompanied us. It made me smile as I listened to them cutting up and acting silly in the back seat.

Justin was invited to go with us on our first family road trip with Debbie and her two sons, Billy and JR. I rented a van and we loaded the four boys in the back for a cross-country odyssey to visit my family in Tennessee. The boys fought throughout the trip, causing plenty of tension for everyone concerned. When I pulled the van into the driveway at the end of the trip, I vowed never to attempt anything like that again.

As he began seventh grade at Grady Middle School, Jake's stomach pain once again flared up and each morning began with a battle: "Jake, you've got to go to school; you've already missed too many days."

"My stomach is killing me," was always the reply. "I just can't go."

We made the rounds to the doctors, searching for medications or therapy or anything that could solve the problem. He underwent extensive testing in the pediatric gastroenterology department at Texas Children's Hospital to determine the problem. Nothing helped. My frustration grew with each passing day.

Finally, I had an early morning meeting with his homeroom teacher to discuss Jake's situation. I told her, "I just want you to know that I'm really trying to get him to school."

Without warning, I burst into tears. I don't know why; I just couldn't stop crying. In between sobs, I managed to say, "I'm just doing the best I can. I promise I'll get him here as soon as I can."

The homeroom teacher was very kind, and sympathetic. "Mr. Driver, it'll be okay," she said.

But it wasn't.

It took all of the energy that he could muster for Jake to make it through seventh grade at Grady. Once again, the end of the school year was an immense relief, and we settled into our usual summer routine – eating out almost every night and going to museums, movies, plays and concerts.

Over the course of that year, we saw some of the best bands in the business, including Credence Clearwater Revival, Peter Frampton, Jimmy Page and Bob Dylan. We also saw Peter, Paul and Mary at the Arena Theatre. These great bands and musicians inspired Jake to work on improving his skills on the guitar, so he began taking guitar lessons at Rockin' Robin, a well-known Houston guitar store that caters to the string musician. He was a quick study who could instantly learn and play the best-known guitar riffs. I was impressed to see that he was gradually becoming an accomplished guitarist.

In the fall of 1997, Jake started eighth grade at Spring Branch Middle School, and his stomach pain continued unabated. On the one hand, he excelled academically. Again, he made good friends and started participating in extracurricular activities. But as the year progressed, he also missed a total of 30 days of school, and this time, the assistant principal was not sympathetic. She met with both of us and lectured Jake sternly about the necessity of attending class.

"We have students at this school who have cancer," she told him. "They endure awful treatments, but they still make it to class, even while they're in serious pain."

Jake looked straight into her eyes and replied: "Who's to say I'm not in more pain than they are?"

CHAPTER 5

WHEN DO YOU KNOW?

*"creation in this world is a product of the soul's doing
expression of the soul is all that matters
we are moving upwards in awareness
always."*

FROM JAKE'S POEM "ONE"

Anyone who has ever parented a teenager understands the challenges of dealing with crazy mood swings, depression, and involvement in questionable activities that could have dire consequences. But how do you know when the problem is something more than typical teen angst?

While some experts estimate that about one-third of children diagnosed with Attention Deficit Hyperactivity Disorder (ADHD) are actually suffering from bipolar disorder, it can take years to receive a definitive diagnosis since doctors are reluctant to label a child or teen as bipolar. Until recently, manic depression was thought to only affect people over the age of 20. Those issues are further complicated by the fact that there are no lab tests that definitively diagnose bipolar disorder and each person experiences symptoms differently. As a result, many children suffer needlessly without proper treatment and medication.

Jake, like most children destined to suffer from bipolar disorder, did not fit the same patterns for the disorder as adults. His mood swings occurred much faster. Whereas, an adult may take weeks to cycle between manic and depressive episodes, Jake was often on a roller coaster, starting the day upbeat and ending depressed or vice versa. He was intelligent, creative and precocious, but he could also be inflexible and throw violent temper tantrums.

Even if they have an awareness of the disease, parents, teachers and doctors often do not recognize the signs of bipolar disorder because they don't all occur at once. Many of the early signs are quite naturally blamed on other events, such as a parent's divorce, or being spoiled and undisciplined.

When you are in a public place and your child throws a temper tantrum, the stares of others seem to say, "Can't you control that spoiled brat?" From experience, I can tell you that no one is suffering more in that situation than the parent who is trying to deal both with their own embarrassment *and* the results of biology gone wrong.

They say hindsight is 20/20, and I now realize that many of Jake's early problems that occurred while living with Anne were probably symptomatic of his disease as was his recurring stomach pain. But at the time, I blamed a host of other factors for the problems and lived in fear that the stomach pain was an awful, life-long disease or terminal illness that the doctors couldn't find.

This uncertainty was compounded by the fact that there were times when Jake seemed perfectly normal. When his stomach wasn't hurting, he spent a lot of time playing his guitar and doing all the things boys his age would normally do. It was easy to forget that there was anything wrong and I lived in hope that, this time, the problems would not return.

Of course, they always did.

Jake was about 14 when we first heard the word "bipolar" in connection with his problems. After a particularly bad episode, he was admitted to Spring Shadows Glen, a Houston-area psychiatric hospital, and Debbie had joined me at the meeting with his psychologist. He told us that he strongly suspected that Jake was bipolar and possibly borderline schizophrenic. Schizophrenia is characterized by both hallucinations, seeing or hearing things that aren't there, and delusions, believing something that isn't true.

After several years of wondering what was wrong, it was somewhat of a relief to finally have a diagnosis for Jake's problem. It provided a glimmer of hope that perhaps something could be done – that effective treatment might finally be had that could help Jake live a more normal life. But like so much of this journey, those glimmers often turn to darkness, and you are quickly faced with the stark reality that your child is sick with an incurable disease.

The doctor suggested that we start Jake on the drug Lexapro to help with the mood swings. There was no guarantee that it would work. He told us that he would prescribe small doses in the beginning. If the medication worked, we might notice an improvement in six to eight weeks. There would be no miracle cure.

That summer, we enjoyed another of our vacations together, this time, traveling to Hot Springs, Arkansas. His friend, Justin, came along, and the three of us stayed at the historic park hotel and enjoyed sightseeing and diamond hunting at a nearby diamond mine.

That was the same summer that the Rolling Stones made one of their legendary American tours, and Jake and I had great tickets for their Houston performance at the city's premier concert venue, the Summit. Hearing great music inspired Jake to resume his guitar lessons, and this time, he chose to study at Fuller's Vintage Guitars, where an instructor specialized in teaching unique guitar riffs.

As he turned 16, Jake was once again living with his mother. She had returned from California about two years before and had rented an apartment near me. In the interim years, he alternated back and forth between staying with each of us. He was doing great in high school, with good friends, and he had both his mom and dad available to him. During the summer, he took driving lessons and successfully passed his driving test. He was excited to have his drivers license and, of course, he wanted to get a car right away, but we wanted him to practice more before that happened.

The biggest event of that summer was our wedding. After seven years of dating, I had finally proposed to Debbie. Our relationship had been on again, off again for the first few years, mostly due to my reluctance to commit to another person after my devastating divorce and my concern about involving anyone in the ongoing drama associated with Jake. It was a lot to ask, no matter how much you might love each other.

But Debbie is a loving, caring person, and through the years, I had come to rely upon her support and strength in dealing with Jake's problems. Since 1996, we had been together constantly, and I realized that she was my perfect match. We shared the same values and had the same commitment to family. I knew that if I didn't marry her, I'd be making the greatest mistake of my life.

So on a beautiful summer day, July 1, 2000, we were married at the Snow Hill Methodist Church near Smithville, a beautiful old church built in the early 1900s on land donated by my grandparents. I grew up on Snow Hill and my grandparents and two aunts and uncles lived on either side of the church. I couldn't think of a more perfect place to marry the love of my life.

My entire family was there and Jake was beside me, serving as my best man. He was tall and handsome in his tuxedo; and he wore a big smile on his face. Debbie looked beautiful as she came down the aisle on the arms of her sons, JR and Billy. Our three sons lit the unity candle together, signifying the joining of our two families.

Jake behaved well during the wedding, and he even performed a loving and moving toast at the reception. But the next day, it was obvious that he was very depressed, and on the way to the airport, the dam burst. We stopped for gas and Jake got out of the car and stood beside me while I pumped the gas. Tears rolled down his cheeks as he told me he couldn't believe I had just married Debbie. I tried to reassure him, telling him that everything was going to be okay, but he was distraught. I felt badly for him because he was so sad that his family was once again changing in a big way.

The downward spiral that began in middle school continued at Memorial High School. On the one hand, some things went very well as he began this new chapter of his journey to adulthood. Memorial is one of the Spring Branch Independent School District's premier high schools, and it allowed Jake to continue his creative interests. He was involved in theatre, performing in a number of plays, and he made new friends through the school's thespians' organization. He was a member of the Class of 2002.

Jake was passionate about music, and he continued to refine his guitar skills. It seemed that there was always a guitar in his hands. He loved the music of The Dave Matthews Band and went to several of their concerts at the Cynthia Woods Mitchell Pavilion in the Woodlands. He listened to Pink Floyd, Tom Petty and Jimi Hendrix and his playing developed a raw bluesy sound. He was talented at making up songs and could improvise new music on the spot. I have wonderful videos of him playing at home and jamming with family and friends. His spontaneous musical acumen still amazes me.

During his sophomore year, he and some high school friends formed a band called "Blue Smoke." For a while they were a popular band at school and played for friends in the Memorial area.

For his 17th birthday, I bought him a used red Jeep Cherokee to make it as easy as possible to go to school. He loved his new freedom and for a while, it actually seemed as if things were going to be better for him.

Then, he just stopped going to school.

"I'm not going. My stomach hurts," he complained day after day. Once again, we made the rounds to all the doctors and specialists. No one could find anything physically wrong.

By February of his junior year, he had missed 69 days of school. The attendance officer called us in for a meeting and told us that if Jake missed five more days of school, they were going to expel him. He explained that the school gets paid by the State of Texas based on how many students they have enrolled and how many days they attend. It struck me that he didn't care about Jake or his problems; all he cared about was getting the school's money from the state. But then, I had already learned that public schools are not equipped to deal with the problems of mental illness. Teacher training related to mental health issues is inadequate in almost every state, and as a result, teachers are unable to recognize symptoms or communicate effectively with students and parents dealing with mental illness.

Jake missed the next five days straight. In fact, he never went back. At 17, his illness had taken a major toll on him and he dropped out of school.

I scrambled to find a school that would take him and help him earn a high school diploma. A friend recommended The Tenney School, a private school that specializes in individualized learning through a one-student, one-teacher approach. His son had finished high school there after having problems in public schools. It seemed like a perfect solution – Jake could get the special attention he needed and best of all, the school was only a couple of blocks from Anne's apartment. He could actually walk to school. So I paid the expensive tuition and he was enrolled.

The first day seemed to go fine. Then, he attended part of the second day, and a few hours on yet another day. But then, we were back to "I can't go to school today." And at the end of two weeks, he said, "I'm not going any more. My stomach hurts."

Later that spring, however, there was a wonderful happy moment when Jake attended Memorial High School's junior prom. Though he was no longer in school, he was invited to attend the prom by high school friends from the Blue Smoke Band. Anne invited me to her apartment, and we snapped pictures of Jake and his friends in their formal wear. Each boy had a date, including Jake who went with a girl from school whom he really liked. We were so proud of him that night. He looked handsome in his tuxedo and he was very excited. It was a great evening for him, and his mother and I were both delighted and relieved to see him have a fun night out with friends.

The moments of normalcy were becoming all too few.

CHAPTER 6

THE LOSS OF LEGAL RIGHTS

*"time will change your body
time does little to change your heart"*

FROM JAKE'S POEM "WHISPERS"

Dealing with bipolar disorder in a child is difficult. Dealing with the disease in a young adult is harder.

Once your child turns 18, you no longer have the legal right to obtain access to medical records. Doctors are no longer required to discuss your child's medical condition with you. Your parental rights have ended, but you continue to be faced with all-consuming problems and mounting costs.

By age 18, Jake's symptoms were in full bloom and the signs of depression and the opposing mania were obvious and lasted longer. During a depressed cycle, he would be convinced that the world was conspiring against him. He would lash out angrily at friends and family and over time, his friends dwindled to just a few.

He wanted his own place. I knew, of course, that this was not a good idea, but at this point, I was becoming afraid for him to live with me. With Debbie and I both at work all day, he would be alone for 10 to 12 hours at a stretch. There was always the possibility that he might become agitated and be destructive or cause harm to himself or someone else. His mother couldn't deal with him. My wife was justifiably concerned to be around him. He didn't have a job. He wasn't in school. I couldn't be sure what he would be doing during the day or what I would find when I came home at night.

After much consternation, I rented an apartment for him in the same complex where his mom was planning to move. It seemed like a good decision. He could live on his own but his mom would be close by in case there was a problem. As soon as I told Anne, she decided to live in a different apartment complex away from Jake.

I moved Jake in anyway and he liked having his own place. He enjoyed having his freedom and, as was often the case when a change was made, things seemed to go well for a short period of time before taking a turn for the worse.

He became depressed. He was always tired and his place was a mess. During these times, I would go over and clean up piles of dirty dishes and sort through stacks of clothes thrown everywhere. I spent hours talking to Jake, doing errands and favors, taking him out to eat, to events and museums, all in the hope that it would help him feel better.

Then, there were the manic periods. Psychologists called this manic, or mania, because the person may be abnormally happy, full of energy and optimism and feel that he can conquer the world. During his manic phases, Jake needed no sleep. He would stay up all night, cleaning his apartment. Everything would be in perfect order. The clothes were hung up neatly. The desk was cleaned and organized. His thoughts would race and he would make lists of all the things he was going to do this week and next month. He wrote his poetry. He painted. He created all sorts of things.

It was during one of these times that Jake decided to get his high school diploma. It had bothered him when his friends graduated in the spring and later that fall, he informed me that he needed money to take the GED exam. I was a little skeptical, especially when I learned that he was required to be there at 8 a.m., but I gave him the money. To my surprise, he called me after the test to tell me that he had passed. He had actually gotten his high school diploma!

For the caregiver, these are the good times – the times when you get false hope those things may actually get better. But eventually you learn that it won't last and you begin to live in fear of the next depressed cycle.

Living alone made it easier for Jake to self-medicate using prescriptions, alcohol and illegal drugs. According to the *American Journal of Managed Care*, 56 percent of those with bipolar disorder have experienced alcohol or drug addiction. Many doctors believe that these individuals turn to drugs and alcohol as a way to stabilize their moods and deal with the alarming symptoms they experience, such as anxiety, pain, depression and sleeplessness. However, alcohol and drugs usually have the opposite effect than the person intends and may actually trigger depressed or manic moods.

I don't know exactly when Jake began to self-medicate, but over time, the problem became obvious. Of course, like most people with this disease, his biggest problem was not drugs, but his inability to cope with the highs and lows of bipolar disorder. He would take too much of his prescribed medications in the hope of feeling better faster or he would decide that he was perfectly all right and would stop taking them altogether. He drank with friends and alone, and he smoked marijuana.

It was a recipe for disaster.

By the time Jake turned 19 in 2002, he had already been prescribed more than 20 different drugs for depression, bipolar disorder and other problems. He had seen at least a dozen doctors – pain specialists, psychologists, and psychiatrists. He had been hospitalized numerous times. And suicide was increasingly becoming a real possibility. But according to the State of Texas, he was an adult and could make his own decisions.

The one bright spot during this period was his psychologist. He had been seeing this particular psychologist for several years and while I was no longer privy to what they discussed during their sessions, he would alert me whenever Jake said anything that was concerning. He connected with Jake in a way that few doctors had and he was also very responsive when there was a problem.

On one particular night, I was driving to the airport for a business trip when Jake called me. He was very distressed. I notified the doctor, and he called Jake and talked him through the crisis.

At some point after Jake turned 18, the doctor and I had a very frank discussion that left me strongly aware of what the future held. "This is not a short-term illness and things are only going to get worse," he told me bluntly. "You are going to be taking care of Jake for the rest of your life."

It was time to get prepared.

The financial burden of Jake's illness was beginning to weigh heavily. Between paying for his living expenses, apartment, food, medications, doctors and especially hospital stays, the bills were non-stop. And I was still paying the price for a financially devastating divorce. While Debbie and I were now a two-income family and Jake was covered under our

Chevron insurance, the uncovered portion was substantial and I was left with huge bills. Anything would help.

During one of Jake's hospital stays, someone had told me that Jake's disability might make him eligible to receive Social Security benefits. I researched Social Security and determined that Jake was, indeed, eligible. While it wasn't a great deal of money, it would be a big help with his monthly expenses.

I explained to Jake what we were going to do, and he agreed to go to the Social Security office with me. We filled out the forms and sat down to talk with a very nice lady. Just as I thought everything was going to go smoothly, she asked Jake to sign a piece of paper. He burst into sobs.

Embarrassed, I asked the lady to excuse us for a moment. She was very kind, and said, "Oh no. That isn't necessary. We're about through here. Just sign this and we're done." The whole process took about five minutes, and Jake began receiving benefits a few weeks later.

CHAPTER 7

WARNING SHOTS

"the time has come,
now buy me a dream
there's nothing more to say
i bought this world
i bought a boat,
and now i'll sail away"

FROM JAKE'S POEM "2786"

The emotional roller coaster that families must ride when dealing with bipolar disorder is frightening enough, but living with the constant fear that your child may choose to end his own life is even worse.

Suicide is the third-leading cause of death in adolescence and some experts have reported that children as young as five or six years old have made suicide attempts. But it is one thing to read those statistics and an entirely different thing to experience it with your own child.

By 2002, suicide had become a recurring theme with Jake. Like many parents of children with mental illness, we didn't take him seriously when he first began to talk about killing himself. It was inconceivable that an intelligent young person who was so loved and with so much promise and life ahead of him could want to end it. But as time went on, the threat became increasingly real and alarming.

Jake's preoccupation with death seemed to grow with each passing year. And just as we were beginning to become deeply concerned about this threat, tragedy struck from a different direction. Debbie's 22-year-old son, JR, was killed in a motorcycle accident.

It seemed so senseless. He was attending a motorcycle rally at a state park near Lake Somerville when a guy he had met there offered to let him take his Harley-Davidson for a spin. JR had ridden motorcycles but not a Harley, so he was excited at the offer. Just as he was getting on, a young woman told him that she had never ridden on a Harley and asked if she

32

could go along with him. He said yes, and they took off around the park road. On a curve, he lost control of the bike and tried to lay it down. In doing so, he was thrown into a metal post. He died instantly; the girl was injured but survived.

We were all shocked and devastated. JR had left behind an eight-month old son and a fiancé, so there were plenty of problems and details to take care of. Most of all, I tried to be there for Debbie in her unfathomable grief as she dealt with the loss of her son.

Jake was very shaken. It was his first experience at losing someone near his own age that he knew well and he took it hard. He attended the funeral with Anne, and although he didn't say much, it was obvious that he was sad.

Now, we talked more and more about death. "I want to kill myself," had become a common refrain from Jake, and as time passed, he simply said, "I just want to go home." He repeated it often and it was chilling to hear.

While Jake could be violent at times, he could also be very docile and sad. During one particularly bad episode of depression, he came to stay with us. Usually, he wasn't too fond of Debbie, but now, he sat on her lap, hugged her and cried and cried as he repeated "I just want to go home" over and over.

A few days later, we arrived home from work to find that Jake had found and consumed several bottles of wine and beer that we had stored. We thought he was high, and over the next several hours, we tried to calm him down. After a while, he became deeply depressed and agitated. He grabbed a Magic Marker and started to write on the wall and floor. When I tried to stop him, he stabbed me with the marker.

Next, he ran outside yelling and headed to a neighbor's house to write on their garage door. I followed him and tried to stop him, but he kept going. Debbie followed me outside and I told her to call 911. Soon, police cars, a fire engine and an ambulance arrived. I told them what was happening and they devised a plan to "capture" Jake without harm. I helped five or six of these great guys grab Jake and put him on the ground. While holding him down, Jake bit my leg. I still have a scar from that bite. After securing Jake to a gurney, the ambulance took him to Harris County Psychiatric Center (HCPC).

By that time, Debbie and I were shaking all over. After the emergency responders left, we started to go back inside our house. It was only then that we realized that 20 to 30 of our neighbors had witnessed Jake's capture and were standing in the street staring at us. One of them, trying to be helpful, approached us and said, "You know, there are medications Jake could take to keep him from acting like that."

I didn't know what to say.

Early the next day, we went to see Jake at HCPC. The hospital had run all kinds of tests and found nothing in his system. Their conclusion was that his behavior was prompted by something other than alcohol. It was yet another sign of what the future would hold for us all.

It was March 28, 2002, when Jake made his first serious attempt at suicide. We had spent a pleasant evening together, having dinner at Benihana downtown after I finished work. We said goodnight and nothing seemed amiss.

Around one o'clock in the morning, my phone rang. It was the Houston Police – Jake had been in a serious automobile accident. He had crashed his Jeep Cherokee head on into a bridge abutment. Thanks to the seatbelt and airbag, he wasn't seriously injured, but his car was a total loss.

At first, everyone assumed that he had taken the curve too fast or had lost control, but after investigating, the police officer told me that it looked as if Jake had driven into the abutment head on without braking. I said nothing, but inside, my heart sank and I thought, "Yes, that fits."

Only two days later, he tried again. I was traveling on business when Jake called to tell me that he was about to kill himself. His mother received the same call. Anne rushed to Jake's apartment and he refused to let her in. As she stood outside his door, he repeatedly told her that he was going to kill himself. She tried to reason with him, but as time passed, she became more and more frightened.

"What do I do?" she sounded frantic over the phone.

"All you can do is call the police and get help," I said, feeling scared and helpless.

The police came and attempted to talk to Jake with no result. Finally, they took the door down and transported him to HCPC. Once there, he was assigned a psychologist who made an evaluation and released him to Cypress Creek Hospital.

A few days later, we had a family meeting with the hospital staff. It did not go well. Jake was being difficult; he wouldn't accept help. He believed nothing was wrong with him. It was everyone else who had the problem. It was obvious that nothing was going to change anytime soon. He was discharged a week later with a prescription for Adderall, which is primarily used to treat Attention Deficit Hyperactivity Disorder.

After the suicide attempt, the apartment complex would not allow Jake to return, so I had to find another place for him to live. I finally found an apartment on a city bus route near the Astrodome. By this time, I was taking time off work almost every day to deal with Jake's problems, and since he no longer had a car, it was helpful to have access to public transportation for some of his appointments.

The ominous cloud of suicide loomed over all of us who knew and loved Jake. Even his doctor, who had worked diligently with him for several years, told me candidly that it was not a matter of *if* Jake would commit suicide but *when*.

I dreaded each phone call.

One day, the manager of Jake's apartment complex called and said there was an emergency. Jake was in her office and had told her that he had taken too many prescription pills and was worried. I took off immediately to pick him up and take him to an emergency room. Luckily, he was okay.

Pressing him on why he took too many pills, he told me that he wanted to go to West Oaks Hospital. That seemed a little strange except for the fact that he had met some of his best friends at West Oaks and he found comfort in being there. To him, it was a safe environment with people his own age, many of whom had similar problems.

Off and on, over several years, Jake spent many months at West Oaks, and it was during one of his stays that he met Beth who would become his first and only serious girlfriend. He and Beth got along well and eventually started dating and even lived together for a while. In reading his poetry, it is obvious that his time with Beth was one of the best periods of Jake's life.

Beth seemed like a nice girl and she adored Jake. She was cute, smart and had earned a degree in child psychology. She drove a new BMW. She worked for Child Protective Services and was at West Oaks to address depression caused by the unbelievable child abuse she saw on a daily basis. It seemed like a miracle that finally, Jake would have someone to talk to, socialize with and spend time with besides me. Things seemed to go fairly well for several months.

But even falling in love couldn't solve Jake's problems.

SUICIDE BY POLICE

"i am fearful, i am very very fearful of what i will do next
i have an open flesh wound,
i'm in a white room,
with a tiny cross the size of a plus sign.
it smells of antiseptic and me
seems i have placed little effort into eternity
i must contemplate it quickly"

FROM JAKE'S POEM "NOW YOU KNOW"

Fifty percent of Americans killed by police each year have a mental illness. It is an appalling statistic that underscores the misinformation and stigmatization that often surround mental illness in our criminal justice system. Yet, only ten percent of the more than 25,000 police departments in the U.S. require crisis intervention training that teaches officers how to identify and effectively deal with the mentally ill.

Nearly half a million people with severe psychiatric disorders are incarcerated in America's jails and prisons. According to a study by the Justice Department, over half of the inmates in U.S. prisons have mental health problems; however, thanks to a severe shortage of psychiatric beds, jails have no choice but to accept the mentally ill patients delivered by police. A 2010 study by the National Sheriffs' Association and the Treatment Advocacy Center found that, nationwide, more than three times as many mentally ill people are housed in prisons and jails as in hospitals. While in jail, they receive little or no treatment, which only makes their problems worse, and they are more likely to be preyed upon or injured in a fight while in jail.

If you have a child who suffers from bipolar disorder, you are almost certain to encounter the police and the criminal justice system at some point. In Jake's case, these encounters occurred with increasing frequency as his disease progressed. By 2003, there had already been several situations that involved law enforcement, but nothing could have prepared me for Jake's attempt to commit suicide by police.

After they had been dating a while, Beth's mother wanted to meet Jake's family. So on February 23, 2003, she and Beth came to our house. We had a nice visit together and Jake behaved like a gentleman. I think Beth's mom left feeling fairly satisfied that Jake came from a nice family.

After our visit, I started to drive Beth and Jake back to his apartment. I had refused to buy Jake another car after he wrecked his Jeep Cherokee, and Beth had recently had an accident in her BMW. She was looking for a new car, so we decided to stop at a used car dealership to see what was available.

As we drove, Jake became increasingly agitated. He began yelling and behaving strangely. When we stopped at the car dealership, he got out and started jumping on top of the cars. He bounced from hood to hood and was talking in an endless stream of babble. It was obvious that we needed to leave and get him home.

I herded him into the backseat of the car and Beth sat up front with me. For some reason, he grabbed a clipboard I had in the car and began hitting me over the head with it from behind. It was so bad that I was forced to pull over.

"Jake, you're going to have to get out of the car," I told him. "I can't drive like this. You're going to cause me to have a wreck."

It was one of those awful times that caregivers are forced to deal with when you must make a decision about how to protect yourself and others as your loved one spirals out of control. When a person with a mental illness commits violence, it is most often a family member who is the target and it is critical that you know when to take the necessary actions to protect yourself and your family.

On this particular afternoon, we weren't terribly far from his apartment, and I felt it would be safer for Jake to walk home than to continue to drive with him hitting me. We were near the 610 West Loop in the Meyerland area when Jake got out. I then pulled into a restaurant parking lot with Beth to collect my wits. Beth and I began talking about what had just happened. A half-hour into our conversation, my cell phone rang. It was the Houston Police.

"Sir, your son has been shot," the officer told me.

I hurried to the site of the shooting near where I had just left Jake, and when I arrived, the scene was roped off. Jake had already been taken by ambulance to Ben Taub, Houston's leading trauma hospital. The police began to question me, asking who I was, who Jake was and why he was jumping in front of cars. They wanted a lot of information from me, but the only thing they would tell me about Jake was that he had been shot. They didn't know if he was dead or alive. They told me I would have to go to the hospital to find out about his condition.

Later, I pieced together the story of what had happened. After Jake got out of the car, he made his way to the freeway where he began jumping in front of cars. Drivers had to swerve out of the way to avoid hitting him. The Houston Police received calls from several drivers saying that a man was trying to commit suicide. The police responded and stopped traffic on the freeway. No one with experience in dealing with the mentally ill or with training in crisis intervention was called, even though it was a response to a suicide attempt.

The policemen said they approached Jake with their guns drawn. "Hey, what are you doing?" they yelled at him.

They said Jake started running toward them. He was screaming, "Kill me! Kill me! I want to die."

They backed up, telling him, "No! Don't come any further. Back up!"

Once again, Jake yelled, "Kill me! Kill me!"

They shot him in the stomach.

During the ensuing investigation, one of the police officers reported that Jake had found a small screwdriver in the grass beside the road and was raising the newly-found screwdriver in a stabbing motion as he ran towards them. That action, said the officer, gave the police at the scene probable cause to believe that Jake was threatening them with a lethal weapon. They "had no choice but to shoot him."

I was, and still am, highly skeptical of this explanation. For Jake to have looked down at that moment, at that place, and to have found a screwdriver simply lying by the road seemed unlikely to me. Even if Jake had found a screwdriver, the police clearly had no plan of action. There was no coordination, discussion, expectation or plan for confronting someone who was trying to commit suicide and might not be cooperative. There was no effort to talk him out of it. A Taser was not used to stop him. Instead, the

Houston Police responded to a man trying to commit suicide by shooting him. Sadly, this is often the most common response by police in America to dealing with a person with mental illness in a serious situation, no matter how much training officers have.

Today, the police are both respected and feared. We all rely upon the police to keep order and protect us. We don't think twice about calling them if a need arises. In fact, the overwhelming majority of Americans never have an encounter with police. But for many who do, there are often negative – and sometimes deadly – consequences.

I don't mean to imply that all police officers are out to shoot some-one. But all too often, there are news reports of police officers that seemed eager to use their guns to solve what seemingly are non-life threatening situations. When police officers feel threatened, they are trained to protect themselves at all costs. They also expect all citizens, including those with mental illness, to obey police officers' commands without question. When they don't, there are bound to be serious consequences, and even death.

Such was the case with Jake.

Not knowing whether Jake was dead or alive, Beth and I rushed to Ben Taub Hospital. We were told that Jake was in surgery. I tried repeatedly to find out how he was. They couldn't tell me anything. For hours, we sat in the waiting room trying to get information from anyone who would talk to us.

When the surgery was finally over, the surgeon came to the waiting room. He told us that the bullet had passed through Jake's stomach and out of his back, narrowly missing his spine. It had caused major damage to his intestines. It was a miracle he was alive.

He was in intensive care for days. Then, he was moved to a regular hospital room. When I visited him, I noticed that a police officer was stationed outside his door, sitting in a chair. Obviously, he had been involved in a confrontation with police, but no one would explain why the police were there 24/7. I went to visit Jake every day and I stayed with him as long as I could. Debbie and Beth also visited, as did Jake's psychiatrist. Gradually, his condition began to improve.

When I arrived for a visit on March 1, Jake was gone.

CHAPTER 9

A PRISONER

"so you got the bastard in
the restraining jacket
you got him under your control
you're very impressive and powerful"

FROM JAKE'S POEM "FERTILE INSANITY"

As many as 40 percent of mentally ill patients have been arrested at some point in their lives, and now Jake was added to that statistic.

When I discovered that he had been removed from Ben Taub Hospital, the nurses could only tell me that the police had taken him. Sure enough, I found him in the Harris County Jail, charged with a first-degree felony – assault on a police officer. Bail was set at $20,000.

I immediately went to visit Jake. Nothing is more heartbreaking than to see your child in jail. He was scared and begged me to get him out. I promised him I would.

I set to work to find a lawyer. I researched attorneys on the Internet who had experience with this type of case and found a firm that seemed to have an excellent track record. I met with them and explained Jake's situation in detail. They told me that the case had nuances that were outside their area of expertise. (It was obvious that they did not want to take the case.) They did, however, recommend another attorney who was willing to work with us.

Jake's hearing was set for March 6. At that point, I still had not been able to hire a lawyer, so I went to the courthouse alone.

The hearing was a nightmare. Jake stood before the judge in his orange jail outfit, and the judge began asking him questions. They refused to let me approach the bench. The prosecutor told the judge, "He attacked a police officer, your honor. We plan to ask the court to send him to Huntsville Prison for five to ten years."

I was seated in the back of the courtroom and kept raising my hand to get the judge's attention. The bailiff came over and told me to put my hand down.

"I'm trying to get the judge's attention," I told him.

"You don't talk to the judge," the bailiff told me. "That's a lawyer's job."

When he turned away, I raised my hand again. At last, the judge noticed me and said, "It looks like there is somebody back there who wants to say something. Is that right?"

"Yes, your honor," I stood up.

"Well, get up here," he ordered. "What do you want to say?"

I told him that I was Jake's father and explained about Jake's problems with mental illness. "If you can just lower his bail, I can get him out of here and into a psychiatric hospital immediately where he can get the help he needs."

The prosecutor barked, "Absolutely not! If you let him out of here, we'll never see him again. DO NOT let him out of jail."

I tried to explain to the judge about Jake's illness and how many hospitals he had been in. I promised that if he were released, I would take him directly to West Oaks Hospital for treatment.

The judge relented. "It's obvious that the boy has serious problems," he said, looking at Jake. "So by all means why don't you take him and get him some help."

The judge lowered Jake's bail and allowed him to go to the hospital, however, the justice system moves slowly and the process took more than two weeks. In the meantime, Jake sat in jail. I visited him every day, an effort that took two to three hours each time.

On March 20, he was finally released on bail and admitted to the Harris County Psychiatric Center. Two weeks later, he was moved to Cypress Creek Hospital. He was released after a week and returned to his apartment with Beth.

His time away from the hospital was brief. On Mother's Day 2003, Jake was pounding on our door at 6 a.m. It was still dark outside and Beth was with him. He was carrying a butcher knife. He said he was going to kill himself if he didn't get a car and some money. Beth was in tears. I told her to go home and let me deal with Jake.

I refused to allow Jake into the house. He was holding a weapon, and there was no guarantee that he wouldn't use it on Debbie and me. So we sat together on the front door step for over an hour just talking. Jake was depressed because he was 20 years old and did not have a car. As we talked, I could see the knife tucked into the waistband of his jeans. I needed to get it away from him but was uncertain how to go about it.

At daybreak, I decided it was best to take Jake somewhere away from the house. I couldn't take him inside and I didn't want the neighbors to possibly see him sitting on the curb with a knife in his waistband as they went for their morning walks. Around 7 a.m., I took him to Starbuck's at Westheimer and Post Oak. We sat outside, drinking coffee and talking until noon. The time dragged by as Jake rambled on and on about his problems and all sorts of irrational and incoherent things. I kept trying to think of a way to bring this to a conclusion without anyone getting hurt. It was a difficult situation. Finally, I was able to get the knife from him during a moment when he was distracted.

Around noon, I said, "Let's go get some lunch." We got back into the car and started to drive west on Westheimer. We were turning right, in front of the Galleria shopping center, when Jake spotted a policeman directing traffic. He suddenly announced that he was going to "kill a cop" and jumped out of the car. He ran through heavy traffic across Westheimer. I quickly found a parking place and tried to follow him on foot. After 15 minutes or so of chasing him and trying to calm him down, I asked a security guard at the Galleria parking lot to call 911.

When the police arrived, I told Jake he would have to go with them and that he would not have to go to jail but to a hospital instead. I explained Jake's condition to the police officers, and they told me that they would take him to the Harris County Psychiatric Center on a mental health warrant. Once he was processed there, he could be released to West Oaks Hospital. They explained to Jake that in order to place him in the squad car, they would need to handcuff him. He did not resist.

I watched as the police car drove away with my beautiful son looking sadly out of the back window about to cry. It was not the first time I had done that nor would it be the last. It never got any easier.

All of this was happening while we were waiting for Jake's case to go before the court. In the interim, I had found an attorney who would take his case, however, before he would start to work, I had to write a very large check as a retainer.

At the next court hearing, the lawyer was successful in getting the charge against Jake lowered from a first-degree felony to a second-degree felony. Jake was sentenced to two years' probation. It was a huge relief that he wouldn't have to do prison time. Under the conditions of his probation, he would be required to see a probation officer every two weeks for the first six months. After that, they would meet once a month. At each visit, he had to submit to a drug test and be interviewed by the probation officer.

Somehow, we got him through the first six months of probation. I always made sure he got to the meeting with his probation officer. I would leave work, go pick Jake up at his apartment, drive to the probation office, wait for the meeting to take place, then take him back home. It took several hours away from the office, but there was no other option that would ensure that Jake made his appointments.

Eventually, the probation problems began. I was out of town on business and he missed a meeting with the probation officer. Then, he was 15 minutes late for the next appointment. Now, his probation was in jeopardy. He could not mess up anymore without consequences.

He was also dealing with various medical issues. The shooting had left his stomach and intestines badly damaged and he continued to have problems. On November 5, I got a call at 3:15 a.m. that he was being taken to the emergency room at Memorial Hermann Hospital. He had an intestinal blockage and was in terrible pain. The doctors gave him several types of laxatives and prescribed a clear liquid diet. He was discharged the following afternoon, but it was just another in a long series of medical problems that stemmed from the shooting.

Then, there was another of those calls I had learned to dread. The apartment manager telephoned to tell me that the police were holding

Jake across the street from the complex. He had tried to kill himself by connecting a vacuum hose to the exhaust of Beth's car and inhaling the carbon monoxide. He had refused medical treatment, but the police took him to Ben Taub Hospital anyway. The next day, he was once again committed to West Oaks.

As 2004 progressed, Jake was on increasingly thinner ice with his probation officer. Someone at his apartment complex had been supplying him with marijuana and before long, he tested positive on his drug test. The first time, the probation officer let him off with a stern warning: "Don't you come in here one more time like this or you're going straight to jail."

The next month, he tested positive again. The probation officer called me with the news.

My heart sank. "What do we do now?" I asked.

"There is no option," she said. "We have to go to court. He is scheduled to appear before the judge tomorrow at 10 a.m."

The next morning, I took him to the courthouse. We waited for two hours to see the judge as countless people filed through the system before us. Finally, we heard "next!" and it was Jake's turn.

The lawyer talked to the judge on Jake's behalf, but the judge was not amused. "Let's send you to jail for six weeks while we figure out what to do with you," was his judgment.

So it was back to jail. While he was there, the lawyer talked with the judge and reported that, in his opinion, the judge felt that "Jake simply couldn't adhere to the terms of his probation and probably needed to go to Texas' main prison unit in Huntsville for three to five years."

Thankfully, the attorney was able to work out another deal for Jake. He was sent to the Texas Department of Criminal Justice's Jester Unit 3 in Richmond, Texas, a Substance Abuse Felony Punishment Facility (SAFP).

The attorney told us that Jake would be required to attend an hour-long class each day and would be assigned to work in the kitchen. If he complied with all the requirements set out by the court, he could complete his sentence in about eight months. If he failed, he would be sent to Huntsville.

The lawyer and I had a long talk with Jake and explained everything to him. He said he understood and promised to do his best to comply with the prison rules. My heart broke as I watched them take him away. He was only 22 years old.

In Texas, families are only allowed to visit inmates in a state prison on the weekends and only two visitors at a time are allowed. Debbie and I made the drive to Richmond, just outside Houston, every weekend. My mother visited from Tennessee and had the sad experience of visiting her grandson in prison. One of my brothers also came. It was heart breaking to see this handsome young man behind bars. But what was happening to him inside those walls was even worse. Jake was falling apart.

I began receiving letters from some of the other prisoners. "You've got to do something about Jake," they told me. "He cries all the time. The guards are yelling at him. He needs help."

I got collect calls from Jake at all hours. "I can't stop crying," he told me. He asked me to call his psychiatrist and solicit his help in getting him transferred to Rusk State Mental Hospital.

I even got a call from one of the guards at the prison. "Your son is out here and he's been crying for two days straight," the man said. "He wanted to talk to you, so I'm going to put him on the phone."

"Please Dad, get me out of here!" Jake begged, crying. I tried to comfort him as much as I could over the phone, promising him that I would do what I could. What I didn't know was that Jake was not adhering to the SAFP program requirements.

After several months of this, Jake's problems in prison multiplied to the point that he was moved back downtown to the Harris County Jail. His lawyer was not optimistic. In the court's view, he said, Jake wouldn't do what he was assigned to do in prison. It was very likely that the judge would send him to prison in Huntsville for a couple of years.

As the summer began, Jake remained at the Harris County Jail. Then, on June 21, he was involved in an altercation with a guard at the jail. According to Jake, the guard said something to him and he responded with "yes sir!" The guard accused him of having a "smart mouth." He threw Jake on the floor, broke his arm and beat him in the face with his fists. Jake was in terrible pain and was taken to LBJ Hospital for treatment.

According to Jake and other inmates, the guard was known to be violent. In fact, several other inmates signed a letter on Jake's behalf stating that the man had a history of violence inside the jail. I hired an attorney to pursue information about the guard's attack on Jake and an internal investigation was supposedly launched at the jail.

Eventually, Jake received a letter from a lieutenant in the Sheriff's Department. The short, three-sentence letter said:

"An internal investigation has been conducted regarding your complaint filed with this agency on June 22, 2005. After a thorough review of the facts and witness statements, this case has been cleared as unfounded due to the lack of evidence to support your allegations. You may contact me regarding any questions you have."

That was all. The attorney was delighted that we even received a letter. He told me that in most cases, such complaints never even get a response.

So the guard was not found to be at fault and would not be reprimanded. It wasn't much, but at least I could tell Jake that we tried.

The day of Jake's court hearing arrived. I drove to the courthouse that morning mentally prepared to hear that Jake was going to Huntsville for three to five years. In the courtroom, I strained to hear what was being said, but could hear nothing. Finally, the attorney came back to talk to me and gave me incredible news: "Jake is going to be out of jail in two weeks. He doesn't have to be on probation or go to prison in Huntsville."

According to Jake's attorney, the main reason for the court's decision was that Harris County jails and state prisons were overcrowded and could hold no more.

I felt as though a huge weight had been lifted.

CHAPTER 10

INTO THE VORTEX

"god does not care about your notes
he already knows what you wrote"

FROM JAKE'S POEM "ONE FOR THE JUNGIAN"

Behind every child who has bipolar disorder, there is a parent and a family that is suffering. Watching your child helplessly as he or she is consumed by the vicious problems associated with this complex disease is an exhausting, draining vortex of emotions and events.

You are awakened at odd hours to listen to rants about fictional problems, bail them out of jail, or race to the hospital not knowing whether they are dead or alive. You spend tens of thousands of dollars on doctors, lawyers, medicines, living expenses and favors, all in the hope that something, anything, will help.

During a manic episode, you are insulted, yelled at, laughed at and assaulted with verbal threats. Or you listen for hours while your loved one makes unrealistic plans or discusses their latest brilliant idea. When the cycle turns to depression, you feel the frustration of not being able to convince them of life's possibilities and the burden of sadness and guilt at not being able to do anything to make things better.

In the meantime, the world goes on around you. You have to work to pay the mountain of bills that are accumulating. You have other family members who deserve your time and attention. And you have to carve out enough time to sleep and recharge in order to handle the next crisis.

Most importantly, you feel alone.

In all the years that Jake was sick, I never talked about him at work. If coworkers asked about my son, which rarely happened, I told them about how well he was doing: "He plays guitar; he writes poetry; he's enrolled in college; or he's going back to college." I never gave any specific details. I would change the subject or ask: "How are your children doing?" The truth was just too difficult to talk about.

Plus, it is exhausting to try to explain bipolar disorder and expect people to understand if they have no personal experience with mental illness. On the rare occasion when I would need to mention Jake's mental challenges to someone, I would often be told: "Do you know there are drugs you can take for that?" More often, people would just get uncomfortable with the mention of mental illness and exit the discussion as quickly as possible.

Maybe there are some caregivers who gather support, verbal or otherwise, to deal with mental illness on a day-to-day basis. Other than Debbie, I never found anyone to help with Jake. I was always hopeful that someday, somehow, someone would step forward and take Jake to lunch, or to a doctor's appointment, or just sit and talk with him. It never happened and I honestly can't say that I blame them. I think those who knew anything about Jake knew that it would be a tough job to spend any time with him.

As a parent, it is impossible not to flash back to the days when your child was an adorable little red-haired boy who held your hand on the way to kindergarten. Now, you wonder: How did we get here? Why couldn't we just have been a normal family? How did he morph into the person he had become?

Then, there is the constant stress and exhaustion. You receive phone calls at all hours to hear about another problem with police, landlords, or neighbors. You get phone calls at work in the middle of meetings that force you to drop everything and race off to take care of the current crisis. There are never enough hours in the day and you are always tired.

A perfect example was August 19, 2005. The phone rang at 2:30 a.m. It was Jake. He had been released on parole at midnight and had been given a taxi voucher and the money left over from his jail account (I had placed money in an account at the jail for necessities). There was no prior notice; they just let him go in the middle of the night. After his release, he had taken a cab to a Wal-Mart, where he bought some clothes. Now, he was calling from a Mobil station somewhere on Westheimer.

I had just returned late from a very stressful business trip and was beyond exhausted. I quickly weighed the options of having him stay where he was until I could get there or telling him to go to a safe place.

I told him to take a taxi to West Oaks Hospital immediately. Ignoring my instructions, he walked there on his own and checked himself in. He remained there until September 2, when the hospital discharged him without warning. He called me around 3 p.m. and asked for a ride to the Reid Community Residential Facility, a half-way house that provides temporary housing, monitoring and transitional services for minimum-security adult male offenders. I raced to pick Jake up, and then I read West Oaks Hospital the riot act for releasing him without warning me.

Less than two weeks later, Jake was once again taken to Ben Taub Hospital for his recurring stomach problems related to the shooting. While there, the doctors noticed that his arm and thumb had healed incorrectly from the beating he received from the guard while in jail. They removed his cast and prepared to do surgery. Jake received a permanent titanium plate to fix the fractured arm bone.

It was a relief that Jake was out of prison, but there were still problems. During his time in prison, we had let his apartment go. Beth had moved on and would no longer be there for him to lean on. Now, we were faced with what to do about the future. Where was he going to live? How was I going to take care of him and his escalating needs?

For once, a solution actually presented itself. While Jake was in Ben Taub, he made a new friend, Steve, who was in his early fifties. Steve had been hospitalized for depression and exhaustion. He was a member of popular Houston rock band, and he and Jake hit it off. They shared an interest in music, and they both suffered from some of the same problems. Steve needed someone to help take care of him when he was released from the hospital, and he invited Jake to live with him at his apartment in a converted warehouse near the convention center downtown. They got along very well and lived together for several months.

As the end of 2005 approached, I had to make the difficult decision about whether Jake was well enough to travel for our annual family trip to Tennessee for Christmas. I was aware that the stress of traveling can sometimes trigger an episode, and I was always concerned about taking Jake on an airplane. I had read a number of horror stories about people suffering from mental illness who had been shot by security after acting up at the airport or who had been tackled and tied up by passengers on an airplane after having an episode. I did not want to put Jake in that situation, so I always had to make a judgment call about what kind of psychological shape he was in before committing to a trip on a plane. Because of the issues that Jake was having at the time, I decided that it was best for him not to travel that year. I promised him that we would have Christmas together in Houston after Debbie and I returned from Tennessee.

At noon on December 24, about 40 members of the extended Driver family gathered in Smithville for our annual Christmas Eve dinner. Afterwards, we were getting ready to sing songs and open presents when my brother, Jim, came over and told me that Jake was outside. I couldn't believe it.

It turned out that Jake really wanted to be with the family for Christmas and had borrowed the money from his roommate to purchase a ticket and take a taxi to the airport. When he arrived in Nashville, he got a taxi and took it to our family gathering in Smithville, 60 miles away. The taxi driver waited outside while Jake came in to get the money to pay him. I started outside to pay him, but my brother had already taken care of it.

Jake was in good spirits, and I loved having him there. I was so proud of him for being able to buy a ticket, fly to Nashville and get to Smithville, all by himself. That afternoon, he sang with us and performed a guitar solo of a song he had written. He was fantastic. Luckily, one of my nephews videotaped the performance; it is a video I will always cherish.

By early 2006, Jake's roommate's problems had worsened and his friends needed to move him and assume responsibility for his care. Jake's problems were also getting worse. He was, once again, suicidal.

On Thursday, February 2, I received another of those awful 2:30 a.m. phone calls. Jake had overdosed on his medications. He called 911 and went to West Oaks Hospital. His overdose was something that West Oaks could not treat, and they immediately sent him to Memorial Hermann Southwest. Three hours later, we received a call from the hospital informing us that Jake was in critical condition and on life support.

Debbie and I rushed to the hospital where we met Anne and two of her friends. We were told that Jake might have had a heart attack. Still breathing on a ventilator, he was totally unresponsive most of the day. Late in the afternoon, his vital signs slowly began to improve. Early in the evening, a CT scan was performed to determine if he had suffered any brain damage. Fortunately, there was none.

By Friday morning, Jake had regained consciousness and called me from the hospital. He denied that he had tried to overdose and told me that he had been diagnosed with rhabdomyolysis, a serious syndrome caused by a direct or indirect muscle injury that results from a breakdown of muscle fibers and the release of their contents into the bloodstream. It is usually caused by the use of alcohol or drugs.

After his discharge from Memorial Hermann Southwest, we took all of his medications away from him and started micro managing them, with Debbie putting his pills in a daily envelope with instructions about each pill and what time to take it. I would drop off the envelope to Jake each morning on the way to work. Sensing that he was in a near crisis situation, we once again arranged for him to be admitted to West Oaks.

While there, he met another young man about his age who was having similar issues and they instantly bonded. They were both discharged at the same time and decided to live together. They found a garage apartment near Shepherd and Highway 59 that was within easy walking distance of restaurants and stores as well as the Rockin' Robin guitar store where Jake could take guitar lessons. The boy's mother and father called me and we talked at length about our sons and what might happen next. The arrangement lasted only briefly and Jake's new friend moved back home to live with his parents. We agreed that Jake could continue to live in the garage apartment alone.

Jake's overdose was another troubling episode in his struggle that scared us and left us without much hope for his future. The problems were intensifying and we desperately needed a source of information on options and support. Trying to hold out hope and find some relief from the day-to-day stress and worry was becoming exhausting. There never seemed to be enough time, energy or help to make things better.

With this in mind, Debbie and I decided to participate in the Family-to-Family Education Program at NAMI Greater Houston early in 2006. We had heard good things about the program and thought it would be helpful to learn what others had done and were doing in response to mental health issues in their own families. The free program consists of 12 sessions, each two and a half hours in length, held over a three-month period. The sessions are designed for loved ones of individuals living with mental illness and the teachers are trained family members who provide insights based on their own first-hand experiences in coping with a loved one with mental illness.

The program is full of presentations, discussions and exercises that help you learn how to manage crises, solve problems and communicate more effectively. You learn how to take care of yourself and manage the intense stress that accompanies being a caregiver for the mentally ill. It also provides an opportunity for mutual support and positive impact where you can experience compassion and reinforcement from people who can actually relate to your situation and where you also have the opportunity to give back and help others grow by sharing your own experiences.

The first thing that we learned from Family-to-Family was that we were not alone. We met parents, wives, husbands, brothers, sisters and friends, who, like us, were caring for a loved one with mental illness. Our stories were similar and the challenges we faced the same. We shared what worked and what didn't work. The instructors led us through discussions that opened up new ideas and strategies for us. Before taking the program, we felt alone and isolated in trying to manage Jake's illness. Now, we knew there were people – many people – who were in the same situation, facing the same everyday challenges. It was great to have some camaraderie in connection with this important part of our lives.

In one particular session, the instructor asked each of us to describe, in just a few words, how we felt about having mental illness in our family. When she came to me, I said, "I feel cheated." Everyone in the room nodded their heads in agreement. Cheated is perfect word to describe this situation. We all could have also added disappointed and exhausted.

In another session, our teacher described the stigma associated with mental illness. She told us that we should not say a person is mentally ill, but instead say that the person "has a mental illness." After all, someone with cancer is not called "cancerous."

The insights provided by the program were extremely helpful to us as Jake's problems continued to grow and intensify.

During 2006, there were more hospital stays. In October, he was admitted at the Neuropsychiatric Center at Ben Taub, and in November, he was transferred to West Oaks from the Harris County Psychiatric Center.

At this point, finding a place for him to live was becoming increasingly difficult. He could no longer live in an apartment complex. After his various suicide attempts and arrests, no one would accept him as a tenant. Jake thought the ideal living situation was a small garage apartment, but that was out of the question. It simply wasn't safe for him to be alone. Thankfully, the Harris County Psychiatric Center helped us find Horizon Assisted Living. While Jake wasn't thrilled with no longer being able to live on his own, this arrangement provided him with the level of assistance that he needed while still allowing him the freedom to come and go.

As the problems escalated, it became harder to maintain control over even the mundane aspects of Jake's life. Through NAMI, I met an attorney who also had a son who was suffering from bipolar disorder. She and I talked about Jake's situation, and she suggested that I consider becoming Jake's legal guardian. There were pros and cons to legal guardianship, she explained. On the pro side, it would give me more control over Jake's affairs. His doctors could legally give me information about what was going on with him and I could more effectively handle his business affairs. I could intervene with the police if Jake got in trouble. But, on the negative side, it also meant that he could no longer have a drivers license or vote. I decided that it would be in Jake's best interest if I were able to legally act and speak on his behalf.

Jake did not take this well. Although he no longer had a car by the time we took this step, he hated giving up his drivers license. And voting was a big deal and was very important to him. He enjoyed the political process and studied politics and the candidates before each election in order to make an educated choice. He voted in every election he could. He was an avid reader and had a subscription to the *Houston Chronicle,* which he read every day. He also liked to study the financial markets. He looked forward to investing in the stock market at some point in the future.

"When I get some money, I'm going to buy some stock," he would tell me over and over again. Now, all those things would be taken away from him.

To obtain guardianship, you are required to demonstrate to a judge that the individual is incompetent and lacks the capacity to make decisions for himself due to a chronic mental illness. As guardian, you have the right to examine medical records and to make decisions for the individual. You also assume responsibility for that person, including their financial needs, medical care, legal and personal decisions. It is a daunting task, but by the time this decision is made, most guardians have already assumed those responsibilities anyway. Making it legal just simplifies things.

Unfortunately, it only gives you control over a small portion of the problem.

CHAPTER 11

THE HIGHS AND LOWS

"i know of no innocence greater than love,
i know of no time quicker than purity."

FROM JAKE'S POEM "REVERBERATION"

As 2006 drew to a close, Jake was experiencing the manic phase and things seemed to be going somewhat better for him. After trying several different living arrangements, we had settled on an assisted living facility that provided services for people with mental health issues. Jake wasn't exactly thrilled about it, but it was obvious that he could no longer live alone. For me, it was a great burden lifted to know that he might take his medications regularly, he was getting good food, and most of all, was safe and, for the moment, relatively stable.

After he settled in, I got a Metro bus pass for him and he would often ride the bus downtown to have lunch with me and talk. One day, he told me that he wanted to go to college and he had selected the University of Houston. I went with him to U of H where we talked to the registrar. The counselors suggested that it would be less expensive and easier to start at Houston Community College (HCC) and take courses that would transfer to the university.

He enrolled at HCC and started classes at their downtown campus. For the first week or so, he got on the bus each day and went to class. He seemed to enjoy it and was even picked to lead a team for a project in his history class.

But somewhere around the second or third week, going to class became too much for him. "You know, Dad, you don't have to go to class every day," he told me. A few days later, he said he needed a car; it was too hard to take the bus. Then, he stopped going to class altogether. No encouragement or anything I could say would persuade him or give him the strength he needed to continue. He simply couldn't do it. The hope and dream of getting a college degree was gone. Like so many of his dreams,

Jake's illness was the reason he couldn't get up and go, just as surely as if it were cancer.

Jake loved to travel and he had asked me repeatedly about taking a trip to New York. By December, things were going well enough that I decided to attempt it. Although I usually did things with Jake alone, we decided to make this a family trip with Debbie and our grandson, Brandon, going along. JR's son, Brandon, was six and adored his Uncle Jake and the love was reciprocated. They enjoyed cutting up and playing games together and Jake often did magic tricks for him. Brandon loved Jake's card tricks and was amazed when he would make the salt and pepper shakers disappear at a restaurant.

We left for New York the day after Christmas and stayed until New Year's Eve. To my surprise, the trip turned out to be one of our most memorable fun times together as a family.

Jake loved New York. We went everywhere. On Times Square, we met up with Spiderman and the Naked Cowboy, and we spent hours in the Disney, M&M and other stores. We shopped at Macy's and toured wherever he wanted to go – the top of the Empire State Building, Central Park, Broadway – and had dinner at the world famous Lombardi's Pizza at 32 Spring Street.

The highlight of the trip was on a chilly winter afternoon in Central Park. There was a tribute to John Lennon taking place in Strawberry Fields and a musician was playing Lennon's music on the guitar. During his break, he and Jake struck up a conversation, and before long, he handed Jake the guitar. Jake started to play and his skill was obvious as he performed several of Lennon's best-loved songs. Soon, a crowd gathered, applauding enthusiastically as he finished each number. Some of them even gave him money. Jake was on top of the world.

From Strawberry Fields, we walked until we found the statue of Samuel F. B. Morse, the inventor of the wireless telegraph and Morse code. After he got his amateur radio license, Jake had written a paper about Morse for school, and years earlier, he had viewed some of the portraits of famous people painted by Morse in the National Gallery of Art in Washington, D.C. Now, we admired Morse's statue at the Inventors' Gate entrance to Central Park at Fifth Avenue and 72nd Street.

Back at the hotel later that night, things were a little more difficult. Jake and I were sharing a room and Debbie and Brandon were staying in another room a couple of floors up. As often happened during the manic phase, Jake couldn't sleep. He was talking constantly and jumping from one activity to the next. I was tired, and finally, I told him that I was going to Debbie and Brandon's room to get some sleep.

Around 1 a.m., the phone rang. Jake sounded frightened: "Dad! I need you to come down here and bring me some money or they're going to hurt me!"

"Jake, where ARE you?" I was groggy from sleep and confused. I had just left him safe in the hotel room only a short time before.

It seemed he had gone to a strip club near Times Square and had enjoyed several lap dances. Jake was not very worldly, and he naively thought the girls were dancing for him because they liked him. He didn't have much money, and when he couldn't pay, they threatened to hurt him.

I jumped out of bed, dressed and hurried over. As I was walking towards Times Square, Jake called again to say they were going to hurt him if they didn't get paid. I told him to put whoever was making the threats on the phone so I could tell them I was coming. Instead, he hung up.

Just as I was crossing Times Square, I saw Jake walking towards me. I called out to him. They had let him go – he wasn't sure why. But they told him to leave and never come back. Crisis averted!

As 2007 began, the manic phase that had carried us through the New York trip was waning and things were once again rocky for Jake. On January 24, Jake was in his room at the assisted living facility when another resident stopped by to visit. Jake had a coffee pot in his room and the other resident wanted a cup of coffee. Somehow, the conversation escalated and before long, Jake pulled out a fake gun and announced that he was going to kill himself. The man alerted the caregivers who called 911 and the facility was placed on lockdown.

Jake somehow managed to run away and was captured a short time later by the police. He was charged with making a terrorist threat (apparently because he had pretended to pull a gun in a mental health facility). Thanks to the fact that I was his legal guardian, we were able to obtain Jake's release when his Probable Cause Hearing was held in April, but he was not allowed to return to the facility. Once again, we had to find a new place for him to live.

At Easter, Debbie and I flew home to Tennessee to visit my family. We returned to find Jake in Riverside Hospital. When I picked him up, he was slurring his speech and drooling and collapsed in the parking lot. He said he had had a seizure.

I was so concerned about Jake's condition that I drove him to the emergency room at Memorial Hermann where he was admitted. A few days later, the doctor told us that Jake had some muscle breakdown and various other issues but that he was medically stable. He was suffering from depression; he had slurred speech and drooling, but a CT scan found nothing organic that was causing those problems.

While he was in the hospital, I scrambled to find a new place for Jake to live when he was released. Someone at Memorial Hermann suggested an assisted living center in the Heights area near downtown Houston that was more homelike than most facilities. The man who owned it had several houses that he had divided into apartments where he allowed people with various mental and physical disabilities to live. Jake would have his own room, meals would be provided, and he would receive assistance with his medications. Most importantly, he would have someone to talk to – he wouldn't be completely alone. When he was released on April 16, I drove him there directly from the hospital.

The man who ran the facility was very helpful and had a great deal of experience in dealing with mental illness and substance abuse issues. To eliminate the need for giving Jake large amounts of cash, he suggested that I provide him with gift cards to neighborhood places such as Starbucks and Subway where he could go out occasionally.

The house was a lovely old Victorian home and Jake settled into a nice room on the first floor. He had his own phone, a small refrigerator, television and a computer. He covered his walls with maps, and his shelves were filled with compasses, amateur radio equipment and his favorite art pieces.

He seemed to like the arrangement well enough. There was a coffee house nearby and Jake played his guitar there often. He made a few friends who were musicians and went with them to various venues to play his guitar. He started painting again and continued to write poetry and produce creative pieces of art. We made many trips to Texas Art Supply for canvasses, paint brushes and different media. Often, he would look at mundane objects, such as a lamp or a bicycle, and visualize how to turn them into unique pieces of art. He spent a lot of time at the local library where he was an avid reader of current events, especially politics.

At this stage, another meltdown was never far away, and in September, Jake went off the deep end when his computer was stolen. He had carelessly left the door to his room open and stepped outside. He had not locked down his computer as we had agreed. Some of the residents told Jake that they had seen a man named David take the computer. Jake flew into a rage and retaliated by smashing the windshield of David's car. When I confronted David about the computer, he didn't try very hard to deny it, so I suspected that he was the culprit. But in a situation like this, any action that you take may trigger a worse crisis, so I let it go and bought Jake another computer.

The schizophrenic side of Jake's illness was becoming increasingly apparent and in the summer of 2008, he began a series of disturbing psychotic episodes. On June 30, I received a call from the manager telling me that I needed to come as soon as possible. Jake had broken out windows and had threatened him and another person with a pair of scissors. The police were on their way.

When the police arrived, they called the mental health unit. In the end, they had to knock down the door to get to Jake. Once again, he was taken to the Harris County Psychiatric Center where he was stabilized. On July 4th, he was transferred to Cypress Creek Hospital, but he continued to be belligerent and uncooperative.

Two days later, his meds began to take effect and I received a call from Jake asking for food and cigarettes. He was discharged on July 7 and returned to the facility in the Heights. The next day, he complained that he was having a bad reaction to a shot he had received in the hospital. He was taken to Doctors Hospital but was released when they could find nothing wrong.

Interestingly, as Jake's problems worsened, his love of amateur radios seemed to grow. Over the years, he had acquired several pieces of equipment, including Yaesu VX-5 and Icom 207 transceivers. He studied hard for his General Class license and when he passed the test, I bought him a Yaesu FT-857, a small but powerful mobile transceiver. He loved to build amateur radio equipment and one of his favorite pieces of equipment was a Vectronics 20 meter CW QRP transceiver, which he built himself. We had great fun working together to build and install vertical, ground plane and dipole antennas that allowed him to extend his reach and talk to other amateur radio operators all around the world.

By this point, Jake had either alienated or had withdrawn from most of his friends and he was very lonely. I believe the radios were therapeutic for him, providing an anonymous connection to friendly, non-judgmental people who knew nothing about his problems. I often heard him talk to other amateur radio operators on his radio and marveled that he was so smart and articulate.

Jake could talk to anyone about anything, usually with great insight and depth of knowledge. In addition to reading the newspaper every day, he had an extensive book collection, was well informed on current issues and was an excellent researcher. When he was involved in legal issues, he researched the matter carefully and would have long discussions with his lawyers about every aspect of his case. He did the same with his doctors, often suggesting treatments and drugs that they hadn't considered but agreed would be worth pursuing.

And Jake could be quite the dresser. We made many trips to the Gap and other stores for the latest shirts, pants, shoes and belts. Always slim, I sometimes thought he could have been a male model. He was clean shaven about half the time, but the other half, he had a mustache, goatee, beard or long sideburns. I was often surprised and delighted to see him trying different looks and looking so good.

Over and over, I wondered why his intelligence could not have been channeled in a more positive direction. With his talent, good looks and aptitude, he could have been anything he wanted to be. Why did this brilliant mind have to be wasted by such an insidious disease?

CHAPTER 12

GOING HOME

*"i release my wicked smile, i no longer need an ego grin
i smile upon you, i smile in wholesome heaven"*

FROM JAKE'S POEM "ME NO MORE"

The statistics regarding suicide in America are daunting. Suicide is one of the leading causes of death in the U.S. In fact, more people die by suicide than by homicide.

But while the homicide rate has dropped by 50 percent since the early 1990s, the suicide rate is growing. In 2003, the suicide rate was 10.8 per 100,000 people; in 2013, it was 12.6.

For those suffering from mental illness, the probability of suicide is even higher. More than 90 percent of children who die by suicide have one or more mental disorders. About 45 percent of people with bipolar disorder try to take their own lives at some point, and 60 percent of those who succeed were abusing drugs or alcohol at the time.

Then, there are the families. For every person with this disease who is considering suicide, there is a family that is alternating between denial and fear. On one hand, they cannot comprehend how their loved one could contemplate ending his or her life. On the other hand, they live in terror that the next phone call will be the one they so dread.

Early 2009 found Jake in a fairly good place. He was comfortable in the pretty Victorian house in the Heights. I stopped by often to give him small amounts of money and gift cards for extra food and incidentals. I took him shopping for groceries, so he always had a good supply of snacks and treats. Over time, he gradually withdrew from eating with the other men, and he usually ate out or alone in his room.

He had a cell phone, cable TV, a computer and his amateur radios that provided a connection to the world and a Houston Metro bus pass that allowed him to travel around the city. Still, he was always in need of money. Each time I visited, I gave him $20 or $50, but he spent it quickly and always wanted more. I hesitated to give him more for fear he would spend the money on alcohol.

In early January, I was shocked to learn that his desire for more money had inspired him to get a job. He had gone from place to place downtown where "help wanted" signs were posted and had been hired at a Chinese buffet restaurant on Travis Street, not far from my office. He worked the lunch rush, bussing tables and getting drinks. He didn't make much money – probably $10 to $15 a day in pay, and that much in tips – but he had actually gone and gotten the job himself without help from anyone. It seemed like a miracle.

On my birthday at the end of January, I went to the restaurant for lunch. He gave me a birthday card and had made a picture for me. I told him how proud I was of him and I meant it from the bottom of my heart. I took a photo of him with my iPhone. It was the last picture I ever took of Jake.

A couple of weeks later, I went to the restaurant again for lunch, and after I finished eating, Jake followed me outside to smoke a cigarette. He ended up walking with me all the way back to my office. As we walked, he kept talking and I kept asking him if he needed to get back to work. He didn't respond or acknowledge my question. A few days later, the restaurant owner let him go.

At the end of February, we celebrated his 26th birthday at a small restaurant on Heights Boulevard near his house. We had a good time together and he was delighted with the Apple iPod Touch that Debbie and I had purchased for his birthday present.

After he lost his job, the downward spiral into depression began again. Darkness was setting in, and this time, it seemed even worse than before. When I visited him, I could see nothing but sadness and low self-esteem in his face. His room was horrible – dirty with clothes lying around everywhere. He was shaking and nervous every time I saw him. There was nothing good in his life, he said. I have never seen a more depressed person.

The manager of the house where Jake lived alerted me that he was drinking whenever he could get his hands on alcohol. Once again, he cautioned me not to give Jake large amounts of cash since it would be spent on booze.

It is well documented that individuals with bipolar disorder are at inordinately high risk of becoming addicted to alcohol and drugs, and Jake was self-medicating with both. Most researchers believe that they are either self-medicating to calm the anxiety of depression or to prolong the highs of mania. Either way, it only makes the problems worse.

On his good days, when he was manic, Jake was passionate about his new business interests. He had ideas for several small businesses and was avidly pursuing one that would help artists obtain copyrights for their creative works. We spent hours talking about strategies for this endeavor and I bought him several books on developing business plans. To my amazement and delight, he read them carefully and wrote a well-thought-out business plan.

As Mothers' Day weekend 2009 approached, I felt that I needed to visit my mother in Tennessee. She had had a stroke and was now in a nursing home. I knew I shouldn't let Mothers' Day pass without spending time with her, but as always, I was concerned about leaving Jake behind in Houston. Before we left, I stopped by his place for a visit. He had gone out, and I didn't get to see him, but I dropped off a little money and a Subway gift card so that he could go out to eat while we were gone.

When we returned on Sunday afternoon, I knew I should see Jake on my way home from the airport, but I also felt badly that Debbie had spent her Mothers' Day weekend visiting my mom. This was always a sad day for her since the death of her son, and I decided to take her out to dinner and wait until the next day to see Jake.

Monday was a crazy day at work. I was preparing for an offshore media tour for ABC's evening news anchor and there were many details to finalize before we flew to New Orleans on Wednesday. We worked late into the evening, and once again, I postponed my visit to Jake until the following day.

Early Tuesday morning, May 12, I received a text from Jake saying that he was coming downtown. I texted back, "That's fine. I can give you some money."

It was not unusual for Jake to stop by the building. He would often call or text me from downstairs and I would go down to meet him. Usually, I would give him some money and we would talk for a few minutes.

Sometimes, he would get agitated and would start talking loud or act a little confrontational, so the staff at Chevron's building management and security office always kept a close eye on him while he was in the building.

I was in my office around 8:15 when he called. Jake said he was sitting on a bench outside the building. I told him I be would right down.

When I got downstairs, Jake was waiting. He looked terrible – his clothes were dirty and he hadn't shaved in a while.

"Jake, your clothes are so dirty," I admonished him. "You can do better than that. You've got to clean your clothes. I'm going to come by tonight and get your clothes and wash them for you."

"Do you want a cigarette?" was his reply.

"No! I don't want a cigarette," I told him, a little impatiently. He knew I didn't smoke. "I've got some meetings I've got to go to. Let me give you some money and you go up the street and have some breakfast. I'll come by to see you this afternoon."

I handed him $20.

"No! I want $50," he said.

I knew if I gave him $50 he would spend it on booze, so I told him, "No. I'm not going to give you $50. I don't have $50. I'm going to give you $20. Take this twenty-dollar bill and go up the street and get something to eat. I'll come by to see you after work, and we'll talk about more money and whatever else you need."

He was silent. I knew from experience that if I continued to try to engage him, the situation was going to escalate, so I said, "I'm going to go back into the building and get my work done. I'll see you this evening. Go get something to eat."

I turned around. I didn't want to look back because that would engage him further, so I entered the building. The lobby was bustling with people. As I got to the security point, I felt Jake's presence behind me.

"I want $50!" he insisted. He had a screwdriver with him and he poked me in the back with it.

Without thinking, I looked at the security desk where a female security guard was watching. "I think I'm going to need some help here with my son," I said calmly. "He's trying to be a little ornery."

Assessing the situation at a glance, she sounded the alarms, placing the building on lockdown. Jake had just enough time to run out the doors before they locked. A security guard chased after him.

I talked to the guard on duty. "That's my son," I told her. "I gave him $20 so he could get something to eat, but he doesn't think that's enough. He's no harm. It's no big deal. I didn't mean for you to call for help."

But it was a big deal. To Chevron security, Jake was trying to harm me. The police were already on their way.

After experiencing so many situations like this, I naively thought, "Holy crap! Here we go again." But then, I also reasoned that at least they would find him and we could get him under control again. It was obvious that he was going through a difficult cycle.

Since I couldn't leave the building, I went to the elevator to return to my office and await word from Chevron security. Moments later, I received a call from the building manager.

"Mickey, you need to come over to Wedge International Tower parking garage right away. Jake has jumped off the garage."

"Oh my God!" I cried. "How high was he?"

"From the top," was the answer.

The Wedge parking garage is 12 stories tall.

From that moment, I was living in a time warp. What seemed like seconds must have taken much longer but now, years later, it is still a blur.

I raced over immediately to the garage at Louisiana and Clay Streets, but somehow, the police already had Louisiana roped off. There was an ambulance and people around where Jake was lying. There were hundreds of people milling around. The news media was there and everyone from my office seemed to be there. My mind couldn't comprehend how all of this had happened so quickly. It turned out that a number of people from Chevron had actually witnessed Jake's jump from their offices.

The building manager who had followed Jake, approached me. He knew Jake from past situations where he had caused minor disturbances at the office and he gave me the details about what had happened.

The building manager had followed Jake into the garage to try to catch up with him and talk to him in order to calm him down. Jake took the elevator, so he raced up the steps, following the elevator up 12 floors to the roof. He came out of the stairwell just as Jake exited the elevator. He told me that Jake had run straight to the ledge and jumped without hesitating.

A policeman came over to me as I was standing there in shock. "I understand you're the father," he said.

"Yes. What is the status of my son?"

"He's gone. He's dead."

That is how you find out.

"I need you to fill out some paperwork," was next.

I went with him to his squad car and he brought out the paperwork. My hands were shaking so hard I couldn't sign. It was as if I was frozen, yet, I couldn't stop shaking.

Seeing my distress, he said, "Well, somebody's gonna have to sign it."

I guess I must have signed the forms because he let me go. As I walked away, I distinctly heard him say, "Well, I hope the rest of your week goes better than this."

Eventually, I was able to go in search of Debbie. She was working at Chevron's suburban Bellaire office that day, and when the building manager called to tell me that Jake had jumped, I phoned her as I was racing to the scene.

"Jake has jumped off a building," I told her.

"Is he all right?" she asked automatically.

"I don't think so," I said. "Please get downtown as soon as possible."

A co-worker drove her downtown. On the way, she called our good friends, Jim and Mary Boyles, and my brother, Don, to tell them what had happened.

Finally, I made it to the spot where Debbie was standing.

As I located Debbie, well-meaning Chevron employees swarmed around us. I couldn't comprehend much of what they were saying. One person told me that the Public Affairs team would designate a spokesperson to answer media questions about Jake's suicide on my behalf. Someone from Human Resources talked to me for several minutes. I have no idea what he said. Another person offered to help with funeral arrangements. It made no sense to me. A few moments ago, I was talking with my son. How do you go from that to making his funeral arrangements?

Somewhere in the swirling noise, it occurred to me that no one had said the words I needed to hear: "I'm sorry." But deep inside, I understood. People don't know what to say, because there are no words that can comfort a parent in a moment like this. Besides, none of it mattered. Nothing mattered now. All the efforts to save my child had failed.

Jake was dead and my world would never be the same.

THE AWFULNESS OF IT ALL

"i cannot die, it is impossible
i can do anything i want
i'm not even the owner of this vessel"

FROM JAKE'S POEM "REFLECTIONS"

Shock, guilt, denial, anger and depression – those are the normal grief reactions that every website and self-help book outline for parents of children who have committed suicide.

None of those words adequately describe the pain of losing a child.

We had been told years before that it was not a question of "if" but "when" Jake would commit suicide. He had made several unsuccessful attempts, so we lived with the possibility every day. But even with all the warnings, when it actually happens, the reality is overwhelming, the pain is excruciating, and the sadness is suffocating.

Your child is gone.

You are never going to see him again.

All hope is lost.

Nothing will ever be the same.

You will never be happy.

There will never be any joy.

Then, there are the haunting questions that have no answers.

Why wasn't I able to save him?

What could I have done to stop this?

Why didn't I go to his place immediately from the airport when we returned from Tennessee on Sunday night?

What if I had given him $50 instead of $20? Would he still be lying dead in the street?

Why us? Wasn't it enough that our family had already lost one son? Why do we have to go through this pain again?

Finally that morning, I wanted to go home, and I told Debbie that we needed to leave. Not thinking, I started for my car. Debbie stopped me, telling me bluntly that I was not going to drive. She drove us home.

Jim Boyles, my closest friend for over 40 years, arrived at our house. It was a comfort to see him. He stayed with us for the rest of the day, helping us sort through the details as we trudged through the awfulness of it all.

Debbie told me that I had to call Anne. It was a call that I didn't want to make. Having to tell my son's mother that her child was dead was one of the most difficult calls I have ever had to make. On top of that, I had not talked to Anne for a very long time. I wasn't even entirely sure where she lived.

I had to keep moving, so I called her from the backyard as I paced. She broke into tears, heartbroken at the loss of our beautiful son, and we cried together on the phone – two parents who had lost the most precious thing in our lives.

I told her that Jake would be cremated according to his wishes and that I wanted to take his ashes back home to Tennessee for burial. She agreed and asked me to let her know about the funeral arrangements. She said she would try to buy an airline ticket. I told her not to worry; Debbie and I would buy her ticket. She was very grateful.

From her own experience with losing a child, Debbie knew I would need help, and she took charge. She called my doctor immediately. Of course, the doctor's office said they couldn't see me right away, but Debbie would have none of it.

"Look," she told them firmly. "This man's son has just jumped off a building and committed suicide. He needs to see someone. Now!"

They gave me an appointment for the next morning.

The day dragged on.

Jim helped us find a funeral home that would handle the arrangements. The police called. An autopsy would be required. Once the results of the autopsy were received, the case would be closed.

LifeGift, an organ donor program, called, asking if we would be willing to donate any of Jake's organs. I said, "Of course." It gave me a moment of comfort to think that a part of Jake might live on. I gave them permission over the phone, and they recorded my statement. They were unable to take any of Jake's major organs because he had been deceased too long, but they were able to take the corneas from his eyes, some skin and various other tissues.

Sometime later that day, Mary Boyles arrived with food. My brother, Jim, was flying in from Tennessee the next morning. The funeral arrangements were being made. Most of the details were being handled.

And then, it was time to sleep. Of course, sleep is impossible, no matter how many sleeping pills you take. In exhaustion, you finally doze off around 5 a.m., and then, you wake up to find the sadness hanging like a cloud, waiting to descend upon you all over again.

The next morning, Debbie took me to the doctor. She prescribed an anti-depressant and suggested that I begin seeing a grief therapist as soon as I returned from Tennessee and the funeral.

We made a sad little band at Houston's Hobby Airport as we departed for the funeral. Debbie and I, her son, Billy, my brother, Jim, and Anne all flew to Nashville together. When we arrived at the airport, I spoke to security about taking the urn with Jake's ashes on board the plane.

"Oh, that's routine," the guy said.

Routine, indeed, I thought. Not for me.

The memorial service was on Saturday, May 16, at noon. We didn't announce it to anyone in Smithville; it was a family affair. A young minister who lived across the street from my mom had met Jake on several occasions, and he agreed to perform the service. I did the eulogy. I spoke for about 20 minutes, telling the story of Jake's life from my unique perspective as his dad.

Knowing that Jake's eulogy was the hardest speech I would ever make, I made notes on index cards to help keep my mind on track.

I began with: "First, thanks to all of you for being here, and special thanks to my brothers, Jim and Don, for helping me during this time. Thanks also to my nephews, Robin and Bert, for helping us get today's service together."

Then, I recognized Anne and Debbie who were sitting together on the front row and presented each of them with a miniature urn containing some of Jake's ashes.

71

Next, I spoke of how the service was a celebration and recognition of Jake's life. I talked about how much he loved coming to Tennessee, which would now be his final resting place. I shared the story of the 2005 Christmas when I didn't think Jake was well enough to travel to Tennessee and told them how he made his own arrangements and surprised us all by showing up at our Christmas Eve family gathering.

"Jake spent most of his life in Houston, where he loved going to museums and the performing arts. He enjoyed playing guitar and one of his favorite memories was playing guitar in Central Park in New York City at Strawberry Fields. He greatly admired John Lennon, so let's listen to one of Jake's favorite songs."

We played John Lennon's *Imagine*.

I continued by talking about Jake's artwork and how he made art pieces out of ordinary objects such as used lamps. "He did abstract oil paintings, several of which were related to God. And he was working on starting a business to help artists get copyrights for their work. Always an avid reader, especially about politics, he was proud and excited about being able to vote when he turned 18.

"Jake's illness was debilitating. It prevented him from living a normal life, and it eventually took his life. As he got older people would shy away from him, leaving him even more lonely and depressed. Like many people with mental illness, he was often characterized as crazy, a nut case, not all there, psycho, even stupid. So many of us have looked at people with mental illness and have made that same judgment.

"We ask that the next time you are talking to someone with mental illness that you do not rush to judgment. What they really need is for someone to listen to them and try to understand their illness and their pain."

I then read a prayer that Jake had written and asked everyone to pray for Jake whenever they thought about him.

As the service closed, *What a Wonderful World* by Louie Armstrong began to play.

I had dreaded telling my mother, but after the funeral, I couldn't put it off any longer. Debbie and I went to the nursing home, and I told her that

72

Jake had died. I didn't elaborate and I didn't tell her that he had committed suicide. Her tears tore at my shattered heart.

I remembered her sadness when my brother, Randy, was killed in an accident a few years before. She had told me, "I think I'm mad at God." Now, I knew exactly how she felt. I was mad at God, too.

My brother, Don, invited everyone to his house for some family time. It was my first opportunity to talk with Anne about Jake and I wasn't sure what she was feeling. Would she blame me? Would she blame herself?

I was relieved to find that she was very supportive. She thanked me for being there for Jake and apologized for not being there more. In the past few years, Jake's problems had become overwhelming to her and she had made the decision to distance herself. I deeply appreciated her gesture of support.

The next morning, we went to the cemetery to bury Jake's urn. Before we left, I went a little nuts. I wanted the urn to be protected from the soil, so I went to Wal-Mart and bought a waterproof plastic container and put the urn inside. Then, I didn't want the plastic container to get dirty, so I put the container inside a small cooler.

Around 7 a.m., my brothers and other family members stood together with Debbie and me in the cemetery, holding hands. I said a prayer, and Jake's ashes were placed into the waiting hole.

It was at that point that I lost it. Since Tuesday morning, we had been racing around, making preparations, taking care of details. Now it was over. Jake's ashes were in the ground.

I started crying. I cried and cried and cried. No one should ever have to bury their child.

Then, one day in the midst of my grief, my wonderful wife gave me an epiphany. Debbie told me that a lot of people were worse off than me. She told me to think of all the people who have lost a child who was five or ten years old or whose child died at birth. Think about their grief and the fact that they never got to see their child grow up.

"You had Jake for 26 years," I heard her say through my tears. "You could have lost him the first time he tried to commit suicide when he was 19, and even though times were tough, you *did* get to see him grow to be a young man."

I knew she was right. So I wrote a prayer to thank God for the 26 years I had with Jake. I called it my hourly one-minute prayer for Jake, and I said it every hour, on the hour, that I was awake for a whole year:

Hourly One-Minute Prayer for Jake
Dear Lord,
Thank you for letting me have Jake for 26 years.
Thank you for eliminating his pain, depression, sadness,
    heartbreak and hopelessness.
Thank you for making him healthy, happy and perfect.
Hold him in your arms and hug him.
Let him know that I love and miss him every day.
Tell him that when I see him again, we will have fun for eternity.
And please comfort all the people in the world who are suffering
    in any way.
In Christ's name I pray.
Amen
Jake's Dad, Mickey

WHERE DO WE GO FROM HERE?

"and when your hungry son is done
and mass confusion has begun
you'll know it's true,
i was the one
and know i'm through
now i'm just a little voice in you"

FROM JAKE'S POEM "THE LAST WHISPER"

There are no words to describe the physical and emotional exhaustion that a parent experiences in the aftermath of a child's suicide. Well-meaning friends tell you to take your time, grieve in your own way, don't rush through grief. But it is so much more complicated than grief.

There are awful questions to be answered:

Where do I go from here?

How will I ever heal?

How do I face the future?

I had to find some way to fill the first endless days and sleepless nights after Jake's funeral, so I turned to reading. Shortly after we returned from Tennessee, Debbie and Jim took me to the bookstore. I bought half a dozen books on grieving and losing a child and started reading. Those were helpful. It helped to know that I was not alone. I was not the first person to go through this. Nor will I be the last. Everyone who has ever lost a child has experienced these same feelings. It also helped me to understand that this process has no end. It goes on forever.

I will never stop loving and missing Jake.

I went to see a therapist who specializes in grief counseling. She darkened the room, gave me a box of tissues, and we talked. We started with how are you feeling? What are you doing to cope? She told me stories about her patients and some of the things they had done to cope with grieving.

Frankly, I don't remember a lot about grief counseling, except it meant that I was doing something positive. I was trying to make it better. Maybe if I worked at it hard enough, there was some hope that, someday, the clouds would part and the sun would shine again.

"You have a new paradigm in your life," she told me. "You now belong to a very special club – of people who have lost children – and you are not the only member. A lot of things will happen to you in the rest of your life, but you will always be Jake's father, no matter what."

She talked to me a lot about guilt and my feelings of personal responsibility. Guilt, I had quickly learned, is a major component of suicide fall out for those who are left behind. As a parent, you are naturally committed to protecting your child. When your child chooses to die rather than live, you feel like failure.

Like most parents of suicide victims, I believed it was my fault.

If I had given Jake more money that morning, he would still be alive.

If I had retired early from Chevron and taken care of him more, he would still be alive.

If I had taken him out more and done more things with him, he would still be alive.

Of course you know intellectually that it isn't true. But emotionally you fantasize about having done something differently and your child is still alive.

The guilt was made even worse when I finally read the dozens of text messages left on my phone during the weekend before Jake died. Several of the messages from Jake said: "I'm just going to go jump off a building."

How did I not see them before? The guilt became paralyzing.

I shared the texts with Debbie and Anne. They were both extremely supportive. "Maybe God meant you *not* to see those text messages," Anne told me. I wondered if she was right.

In an effort to comfort you, people offer platitudes. Jake is with the Lord. He's not in pain any more. You know it's true. But it just doesn't help.

My psychologist sent me to a psychiatrist. He prescribed anti-anxiety medication and we talked.

"Why did Jake have to kill himself?" I kept asking of anyone who would listen. "What possesses a young person to go up to the 12th floor of a parking garage and jump off?"

"Because of the pain," was the answer. "He could not stand the pain. That's why people kill themselves. If you haven't experienced that kind of pain, there is no way that you can understand it."

"Will this ever get any better?" was my next question.

The psychiatrist drew a big circle on the board in his office with another large circle inside it. "Let's look at everything that is going on in your life right now," he said. "This large circle inside the circle is the part where you are dealing with Jake's suicide right now. He's taking up all of your time, your emotions, your thinking. Everything! There is hardly any room for anything else."

Then, he drew another large circle with a much smaller circle inside of it. "As time moves on and you continue to work on this, as you will, this is where you will deal with Jake in the future." He pointed to the smaller orb. "It will never go away, but the circle will be much smaller in the future than it is today."

He was right, of course. Although, I still think that Jake's circle was too small in the second example.

The people at Chevron were wonderful. I had worked for the company for 33 years and I had taken off almost no sick days. "Take all the time you need," was the message I heard over and over.

I thought about retiring, but I decided that I did not want the end of my Chevron career to be defined by the day that Jake died. Debbie and I discussed it at length and I decided to go back to work and complete two more years so that I could retire with 35 years of service.

During my absence, I did not stay in touch with anyone. My email simply said, "Out of the office until further notice." Debbie kept in touch with my coworkers and let them know how I was doing.

Someone suggested that I start back to work on a half-day schedule. That seemed like a good idea. Someone else suggested that I have a meeting with my co-workers. That also seemed like a good idea.

At 10 a.m. on Tuesday, August 11, three months after Jake's death, I walked into the Public Affairs conference room. I sat at the head of the table with Debbie beside me before about 20 of my coworkers and this is what I said:

"I want to thank you and address any concerns or questions you may have.

"I want to thank everyone for their cards, support, prayers, help, contributions and caring. I know that Jake's suicide has impacted some of you in several different ways.

"I especially want to thank the building management and security team – I know this was tough on you guys.

"Thanks to our Houston Employee Assistance Manager for his help with the company's employee assistance program and his recommendations.

"Thanks to my longtime friends in public affairs who met with Jake's caregiver, cleaned out Jake's room and brought his things to the house. They also brought food to our house and stayed in touch with Debbie and me.

"Thanks to the Human Resources staff for their help and support.

"And most of all, thank you Debbie, my best friend and supporter, who also lost a son when he was just 22.

"I will do my best not to give too much information. I want you to know that I have no problems or issues with talking about Jake, mental illness, suicide, or grieving. But I am not going to discuss these things with you unless you ask me. I understand that lots of folks are uncomfortable with these issues. You don't come to work to hear about them. So don't be concerned that I am going to bring them up.

"If you would like to know more about these things, I have two books I would like to recommend: *His Bright Light* by Danielle Steel and *The Worst Loss* by Barbara Rosof.

"The death of a child is the most horrible emotional and psychological pain a person can go through. It is a nightmare every day; in my case, made even worse by losing a child by suicide.

"I have been off work for three months because my heart and soul were ripped out of me and I have been in critical condition. I had family members staying with me for about two months. Debbie wouldn't let me drive for a month. And today is my first day downtown since

Jake died. I am in grief counseling and seeing a psychiatrist for medication. To deal with the chronic grieving, I am taking anti-depressant and anti-anxiety medication.

"With the loss of a child, you do not heal. You do not get over it. You are changed forever. You are on a journey where you grieve until the day you die. I am just at the beginning of that journey. But you do eventually learn to manage the grief.

"And so, I am starting to slowly move on and starting back to work is part of that process. On my doctor's recommendation, I am starting back to work part-time for the next two weeks, which means I will be in the office four hours a day. I will return to full-time work on Monday, August 24.

"I would like to ask you to not be concerned about talking to me about work. I don't want anyone to be uneasy about talking to me about anything. My hope is to be the same Chevron person I was before Jake died.

"Thanks again to each of you for being here, and again, Debbie and I sincerely appreciate all of your support."

IN THE END, THERE IS ONLY LOVE

*"the world is a breeding ground for love and death
but you're stupid if that reflects your depth"*

FROM JAKE'S POEM "LOGICAL BALLOONS"

The next week after I started back to work, my boss flew to Houston from California to meet with me. Someone else had taken over my job during my absence, so a new job would have to be created for me.

There were several options. He offered to allow me to work half time. I thought about living on half a paycheck and decided against it. I needed a full-time job. He told me that since I worked in the building where I last saw Jake alive and he died just a block from there, I could work from Chevron's Bellaire office. That was a thoughtful gesture, but I decided I wanted to be downtown, near my coworkers and all of our clients.

We decided that I would be an external relations advisor. In this role, I would advise and mentor the public affairs team, something I was doing already as one of the most senior members. I would also assume responsibility for several other areas, including the company's media crisis training program.

I settled into the routine, but there was something that I needed to deal with in order to feel comfortable about being there. A couple of months after I went back to work, I told Debbie that I needed to go to the Wedge parking garage, go to the top like Jake did, and look over the edge from the spot where he had jumped. She adamantly tried to talk me out of it. But I said no. This was something I needed to do.

So we did.

One day during lunch, we went to the garage, rode the elevator to the top, and I walked to the exact spot from which Jake had jumped and looked down. I don't know why I had to do it. I just needed to know what it was like in Jake's last moments.

After that, I was much more comfortable looking at that building from my window every day until my retirement.

Six years after Jake's death, I am still spending a lot of time, energy and emotion dealing with all that happened. I am still sad, and I grieve every day. I often cry when thinking of Jake. But I have found ways to heal.

The fact that the donation of Jake's eyes, skin and tissue may have made life better for others was a great comfort to me. Although the organ bank was not able to use any of Jake's major organs, he was still recognized as a major organ donor. In the year following his death, we attended an annual LifeGift dinner for the families of donors. There were more than 1,000 people at the event and all of the donors were featured in a slide show. There were photos of young children and babies who had died – so many young people, so much sadness, and so many parents who did not have the gift of watching their children grow up.

After Jake's death, I applied for and received the rights to his amateur radio call sign, KC5WXA. In 2010, Debbie, Jim and Mary Boyles and I founded the Jake McClain Driver Memorial Amateur Radio Club to memorialize Jake's amateur radio interests and enthusiasm. We wanted to honor Jake by promoting amateur radio to the general public as a hobby and emergency communications resource. Today, the club has members in Texas, Tennessee and Ohio. It also provides two $1,000 scholarships to graduating high school students who are amateur radio operators. In 2014, we dedicated a memorial bench in Jake's honor at the American Radio Relay League's (ARRL) headquarters in Newington, Connecticut.

The anniversary of Jake's death is a difficult day for us each year, so Debbie insists that we try to be as far from Houston as possible. We have found beautiful ways to remember Jake in new locations around the world.

Debbie continues to be my greatest source of support and strength. When I feel sorry for myself, she points out how blessed we are and how much we have to be thankful for.

Whenever I'm in Smithville, I visit Jake's gravesite, placing flowers, lights and other decorations. I also place flowers and lights on Anne's mother's grave, which is near Jake. The graves of my dad, James G. "Bobo" Driver, my mom, Nell Driver, and my brother, Randy, are also nearby, so

I go and visit with all of them. I look at Jake's grave marker and think about the words inscribed there: "In the end, there is only love."

Those powerful words came from a prayer that Jake wrote and dated February 23, 2009, a few days before his 26th birthday and three months before his death. We found the handwritten prayer among Jake's belongings when his room in the Heights was cleaned out. The prayer reflects a young man's desire for God's presence in his life, and even has a touch of Jake's humor.

Jake's Prayer 2/23/09
I pray for wisdom, for harmony,
for concordance and unity with
all those I come in contact with.
I pray that God's presence will
surround and encompass all that is
being around me and ask the Lord
to allow me to step back and
recognize his influence over
people and places and
things in my life.

Be with me Lord. Open my life
to new directions and possibilities

Help me to understand why
there is a moth on my left sleeve.

For all those I have loved, continue
to love, will always love,
and those I have yet to love
because in the end there is only love

Obituary Houston Chronicle May 15, 2009
Jake McClain Driver

Our beloved and precious JAKE MCCLAIN DRIVER, age 26, left us on Tuesday, May 12, 2009, as a result of mental illness, which finally overtook him.

He is survived by his father and stepmother, Mickey and Debbie Driver, his mother, Anne Bellamy, his stepbrother, Billy Turrentine, stepsister, Holly Beauchamp, and other extended family members, all of Houston. He is also survived by his paternal grandmother, Nell Driver, uncles, Jim Driver, Don Driver, Gary Driver, Terry Driver and aunt, Dorothy Durham, as well as many cousins and other family members in Tennessee.

Jake was born on February 26, 1983, in Atlanta, Georgia, lived in California for several years, and then moved to Houston. He attended Seven Hills School in Walnut Creek, California and Del Mar Middle School in Tiburon, California. In Houston he attended St. Francis Episcopal Day School, Spring Branch Middle School, Memorial Senior High School and Houston Community College. He performed in theater at each school, and was a dual credit college/high school student at Memorial Senior High.

Jake was an incredible artist who played amazing guitar, painted, wrote poetry and short essays. He often performed at coffee houses in the Houston area with his friends. One of his favorite remembrances was a family vacation to New York City a few years ago where he played Beatles songs at the memorial for John Lennon at Strawberry Fields in Central Park. He immediately created a large crowd of listeners with much applause and appreciation of his guitar skills. Jake's creativity and humor were astonishing.

Besides his talent as an artist, he was an entrepreneur who worked on several small businesses, including one to help people get copyrights for their creative works. He was an avid reader of daily newspapers and books and loved conversations on current topics. He was an amateur radio operator, call sign KC5WXA, who thoroughly enjoyed building equipment and talking to his dad and other hams on his radios. He enjoyed attending Theater Under the Stars and other Houston performing arts, and making visits with his family to Houston's art and science museums.

Jake was good hearted, loved his family and friends, and in return was very much loved, admired and respected by them. He would often make pieces of art that he gave to family and friends as gifts. Jake's smile, sense of humor and ability to connect with people made him popular. He had his fair share of girlfriends. He was a very good, decent guy who was dealt a bad hand. He touched many lives and will be remembered always by those who knew him as an inspiration for his courageousness and strength in dealing with so many disappointments and adversities in his life.

The family wishes to express its sincere and heartfelt thanks to all of Jake's caregivers over the years, including hospitals and doctors who spent so much time with him. We are especially thankful to Mr. Lee Castillo in The Heights for his unwavering patience, support, care and love of Jake over the past few years.

We would also like to thank all our family and friends in Houston and Tennessee for your understanding and support of Jake for so long. We were blessed with the care and help you gave us in dealing with Jake's depression and other issues. All who knew and loved him will eternally miss Jake, and he will leave forever an unimaginable void in so many of our lives.

A memorial service will be held in Smithville, Tennessee on Saturday, May 16, 2009, for Jake's family, followed by internment at DeKalb Memorial Gardens. In lieu of flowers, the family would be honored if donations would be mailed to the "Jake McClain Driver Memorial Fund, P.O. Box 55884, Houston, TX 77255-5884." This memorial fund has been established to help support two causes that were important in Jake's life: The National Alliance of Mental Illness (NAMI) Metropolitan Houston, and the American Radio Relay League (ARRL), Newington, CT.

AFTERWORD

It has taken more than six years of tears, grieving and healing since Jake's death to be able to write this story. Even now, putting the events of his short life down on paper is a challenge. Paper seems too flat, too shallow to hold a personality as big as Jake's. And as the story unfolds, it seems that no amount of description or detail can adequately describe the tumultuous events that shaped Jake's final years.

If you have lost a child, you know that the grieving, sadness and sorrow will never stop. You know that others will never understand the pain that can be felt instantly any day for the rest of your life. You also know that your life will never be the same, yet you will somehow learn to live with your loss.

Slowly, we are healing. There are still plenty of bad days. Holidays, Jake's birthday and the anniversary of his death are tough. Every day, there are reminders that he is not here. But as time goes by, there are also good days when we reflect on the joy that Jake brought into our lives and draw upon the wonderful memories that he left behind.

Like many parents who have lost a child, I wanted Jake to have a legacy, for his life to have meaning, and for the lessons learned from his struggles to provide help to others. I understand that no two journeys are alike and that bipolar disorder is definitely not a "one size fits all" disease. Every person has to find their own path and every family has to draw from many resources. But I also understand that reading and studying about the experiences of others is comforting and empowering, and I hope that Jake's story, and his poetry, will help others to understand that they are not alone.

If you are dealing with a loved one who has bipolar disorder, you are in for a difficult journey. There will be times when you will want to give up – when the exhaustion, expense and frustration will seem too much to bear. There will also be times of great love and joy. And those are the times that are worth holding onto. As a caregiver, you are probably doing all you can. Hang in there and don't ever give up hope.

Often, people ask me what I wish I had known sooner and what I wish I had done differently. There are no easy answers to those questions. In the aftermath of Jake's death, there were a million things that I regretted, questioned and wished I could change. Would any of it have made a difference? Would it have stopped Jake from ending his life? The truth is, I doubt it.

The good news is that with proper diagnosis and treatment, those suffering with bipolar disorder can live long and productive lives. Thanks to the advocacy of organizations like the National Alliance on Mental Illness and the work of many dedicated individuals who have traveled this road, there is a growing awareness of the disease in young people. As a result, it is becoming more common to diagnose teenagers and even younger children with manic depression and to prescribe appropriate medications. Bipolar disorder tends to worsen over time if left untreated, which means that early diagnosis and treatment, especially in children, are critical.

It is important to understand that the signs of bipolar disorder are different in children and teens than in adults. NAMI lists the following warning signs of bipolar disorder in children:

Symptoms of mania include:
- Acting overly joyful or silly that is not normal behavior.
- Having a short fuse or extremely short temper.
- Appearing to be thinking or talking a mile a minute.
- Sleeping very little without feeling tired.
- Talking and thinking about sex more than usual.
- Engaging in risky behavior, thrill seeking behavior or over-involvement in activities.
- Hallucinations or delusions, which can result from severe episodes of mania.

Symptoms of depression include:
- Feeling extremely sad or hopeless.
- Being in an irritable mood.

- No longer interested in activities that were once enjoyed–hobbies, sports, and friendships.
- Sleeping too much, hardly ever sleeping or having trouble falling asleep.
- Moving slowly or restlessness.
- Changes in appetite or weight.
- Little or no energy.
- Problems concentrating.
- Aches and pains for no reason.
- Recurrent thoughts or talk of death or suicide.

In our society, people often fear what they do not understand, and bipolar disorder is definitely an illness that is misunderstood. Parents are often reluctant to seek help for fear of having their child labeled as less than perfect. This results in unnecessary suffering for both children and their parents.

So after traveling this road, I have given much consideration to what advice I would like to share with others. Here are my thoughts:

If you suspect that your child has bipolar disorder, don't hesitate to have a frank talk with your doctor as soon as possible. The problem will not go away and it is not a disease that you can walk away from. Your child needs professional medical and psychological help.

While we may all wish for a miracle pill that will cure bipolar disorder, finding the right medications and dosage can be a long and frustrating process. In most cases, it will take some trial and error and a great deal of patience to find the medication, or groups of medications, that work best. Some medications need weeks or months to take full effect and will need to be adjusted periodically as symptoms change. Others have side effects that must be managed. The good news is that medications are helping many with bipolar disorder to cope with their symptoms and live normal lives.

There is much more to the problem than just medicine. This is a complicated, multi-layered illness that will require you to learn to deal with the lack of training and support available from educators and law enforcement and the problems associated with addiction.

There is a surprising lack of awareness on the part of educators when it comes to mental illness. Children and youth spend the majority of their waking hours in school, and staying in school is crucial to their success. Many mental health crises can be prevented if schools, parents and community members know what to look for and how to respond. Schools can start by training staff about the early warning signs of mental health conditions and connecting children who exhibit those warning signs with mental health services.

The problem is equally serious in America's criminal justice system. The sad reality is that while many mentally ill persons come in contact with police – and some 40 percent of people with serious mental illness will be arrested at some point – very few members of America's law enforcement community have had crisis intervention training in which they learn to deal with situations involving the mentally ill. As a result, our jails and prisons are filled with individuals who are suffering from a broad range of mental illnesses for which they will never receive help.

If your loved one is involved in a situation with the police, do not assume that he or she is guilty or innocent. Rather, consider the situation carefully and seek the best help possible. Consult an attorney who has experience in defending people with mental illness and work aggressively to have your loved one released so they can receive proper treatment.

Your support is key to your loved one's recovery, however, the role of caregiver is a difficult one. In order to be an effective advocate for your child, you need to know what is happening in their lives. It is important to spend time with them, take them places, and be there when they need to talk.

It is also important to accept that this is a long-term illness and understand that you alone cannot heal this person. Nor can you take care of him or her 24 hours a day. Whenever possible, accept help from others and do what you must to stay emotionally and physically healthy.

Often when a loved one is diagnosed with a mental illness, we try to hide it from everyone. Would you do that if your loved one had cancer? Probably not. Yet, we are falsely hopeful that the mental illness will go away, and because of the stigma attached to mental illness, we feel ashamed of having the disease in our family. Think hard about the road ahead and don't be ashamed. Mental illness is just as worthy of understanding and help as any other disease.

Not everyone is equipped to handle the problems of a loved one with mental illness. While it can be difficult, it is important to be understanding when a spouse, family member or friend can no longer cope with the problems that your loved one is facing.

Being the caregiver for a person with mental illness has to be one of the most challenging and least appreciated efforts on earth. You sacrifice your time, energy, money and often part of your sanity struggling to make your loved one's life better. Your own health, finances and career can, and do, suffer. I was offered several promotions and international transfers while at Chevron. I turned them all down in order to not move Jake away from his doctors, friends and surroundings that he needed for support. This is what a parent does.

Managing bipolar disorder is a lifelong process. Even when a person is committed to treatment, getting better after a depressed episode takes time. Do not expect a quick recovery or a permanent cure and be prepared for setbacks and problems along the way.

Let your child or loved one know that you love them unconditionally and will support them as they work towards recovery.

Just because Jake's life ended with his suicide does not mean that your loved one's story will also end in an untimely death. It *is* important, however, to be aware of this possibility and to understand that many suicides can be prevented with the right treatment and support. Always take talk of suicide seriously and if you suspect that your loved one is considering taking their own life, don't hesitate to intervene and get them the care they need.

Finally, while it is important that we keep mental illness at the forefront of our social and political agenda, the real battle is fought one person at a time.

Don't be afraid to talk to someone about the loss of a loved one to suicide. Instead of being upset or sad, they will find comfort in the fact that you still remember their loved one and you care. If you don't talk about their loss, it will be like their love one never existed, and that just adds to their sadness and heartache.

And if you see a person who is struggling with mental illness, don't turn away. Don't criticize them. Don't call them crazy. Don't ignore them. Don't move along and pretend that they simply don't exist.

Instead, look them in the eye.

Give them a little of your time and listen to them.

Don't be judgmental.

Give them a hug.

Let them know someone cares.

Let them know they are not alone.

SOURCES

"Depression Health Center." http://www.webmd.com/depression/
guide/bipolar-disorder-manic-depression. Retrieved March 10, 2015.

Faedda, Gianni L., MD and Austin, Nancy B., PSY.D. *Parenting a Bipolar
Child: What to Do & Why*, Oakland, CA: New Harbinger Publications.
2006. Print.

Greenberg, Rosalie, M.D. *Bipolar Kids: Helping Your Child Find Calm in
the Mood Storm*, Cambridge, MA: Da Capo Press. 2007. Print.

Haycock, Dean A. *The Everything Health Guide to Adult Bipolar
Disorder/Third ed*, Avon, MA: Adams Media. 2014. Print.

Hirschfield, Robert M.A., MD, and Vornik, Lana A., MSc. "Bipolar
Disorder: Costs and Comorbidity" June 15, 2005. http://www.ajmc.com/
publications/supplement/2005/2005-06-vol11-n3Suppl/Jun05-2074pS85-
S90/2. Retrieved April 8, 2015.

National Alliance on Mental Illness. (2015) https://www.nami.org.
Retrieved March 10, 2015.

NAMI Greater Houston. (2015) https://www.namigreaterhouston.org.
Retrieved March 10, 2015.

National Institute of Mental Health. http://www.nimh.nih.gov/health/
topics/bipolar disorder/index.shtml. Retrieved March 10, 2015.

Kristof, Nicholas. "Inside a Mental Hospital Called Jail" February 8, 2014. *The New York Times* (Online). http://www.nytimes.com/2014/02/09/opinion/sunday/inside-a-mental-hospital-called-jail.html?_r=O. Retrieved April 15, 2015.

Papolos, Demitri, MD, and Papolos, Janice. *The Bipolar Child: The Definitive and Reassuring Guide to Childhood's Most Misunderstood Disorder/Third ed,* New York: Random House. 2006. Print.

Pinkerton, James. "As mental illness permeates streets, police, jail struggle." January 30, 2013. *The Houston Chronicle* (Online). http://www.houstonchronicle.com/news/houston-texas/houston/article/As-mental-illness-permeates-streets-police-jail-4237636.php. Retrieved September 3, 2014.

Rothkopf, Joanna: "Cops don't know how to deal with mental illness, and it's a huge problem." February 8, 2014. http://www.salon.com/2014/08/21/cops_dont_know_how_to_deal_with_mental_illness_and_thats_a_huge_problem/ Retrieved April 15, 2015.

Serani, Deborah. *Depression and your Child: A guide for parents and caregivers,* Lanham, MD: Rowan & Littlefield. 2013. Print.

Silberner, Joyce. "What Happens If You Try to Prevent Every Single Suicide?" November 2, 2015. http://www.npr.org/sections/health-shots/2015/11/02/452658644/what-happens-if-you-try-to-prevent-every-single-suicide. Retrieved November 5, 2015.

Steel, Danielle. *His Bright Light.* New York, NY: Random House. 1998. Print.

Young, Joel L. MD. *When Your Adult Child Breaks Your Heart.* Guilford, CT: Lyons Press. 2013. Print.

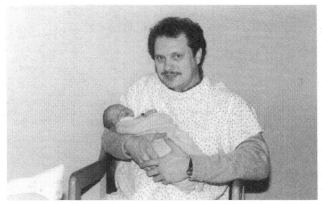

Mickey holds Jake McClain Driver soon after his birth.

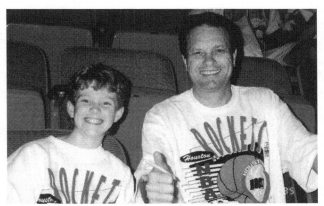

Jake and Mickey cheered the Houston Rockets on to victory during the 1995 NBA championships.

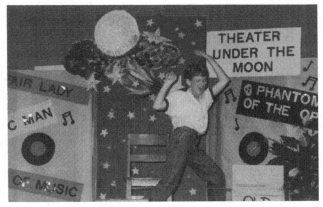

"He's going to be a star one day," the principal told the audience after Jake performed "50 States in Rhyme" in the sixth-grade school play.

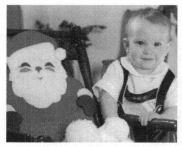

Jake's first Christmas.

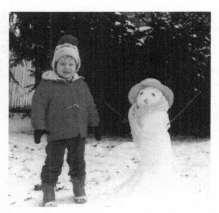

Jake builds his first snowman during a white Christmas in Smithville, Tennessee.

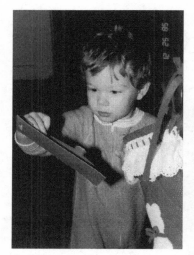

And Christmas #2.

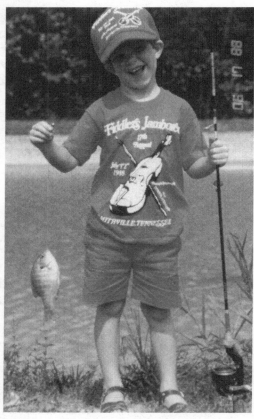

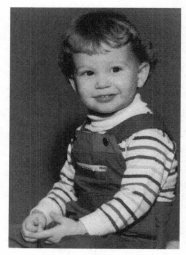

At age two, Jake's red curly hair and impish smile won the hearts of all who encountered him.

Jake was thrilled when he caught his first fish at age five.

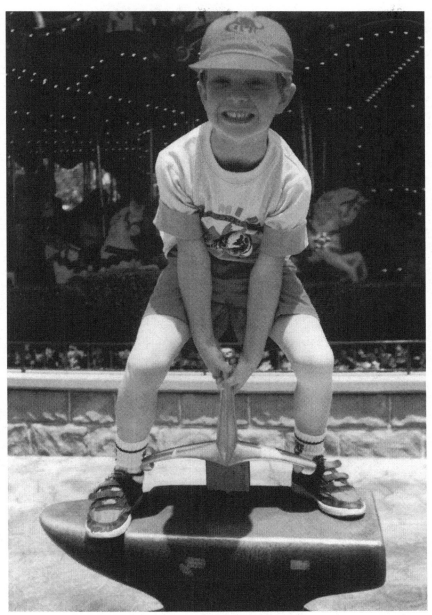

Jake attempts to pull the sword from the stone in front of King Arthur's Carousel at Disneyland.

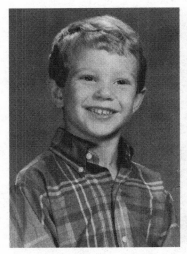

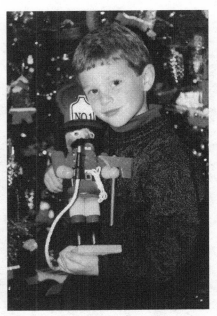

Jake's preschool picture at age 5 shows a bright, happy little boy.

After attending a performance of the Nutcracker ballet, Jake posed for Christmas pictures with his own nutcracker.

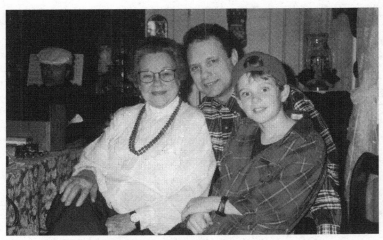

"Mommy Nell" Driver, Mickey and Jake enjoyed spending time together whenever the family visited Smithville.

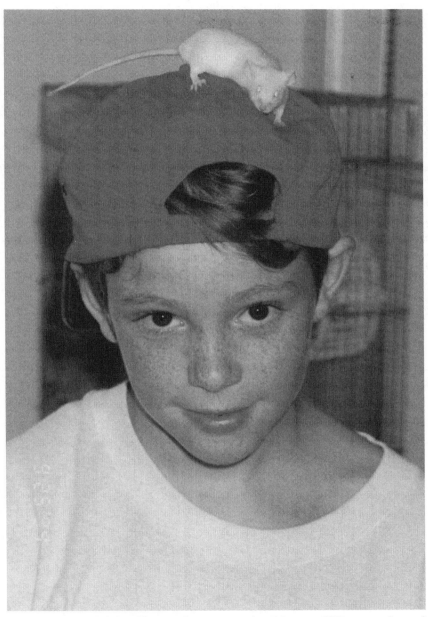

Jake's menagerie included a rabbit named Licorice, two dogs—Cutter and Watson—and several mice. This one was named "Booger."

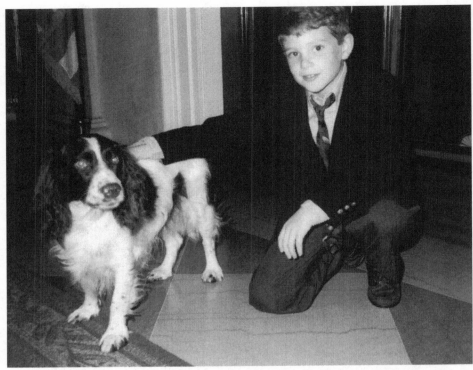

President and Mrs. Bush's dog, Millie, became great friends with Jake during the Driver's White House visit.

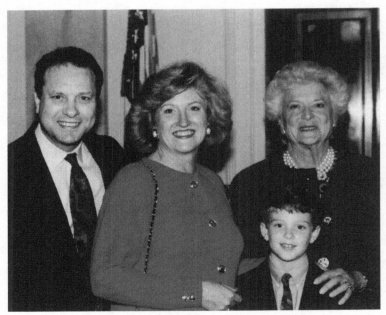

Mickey, Anne and Jake pose with First Lady Barbara Bush.

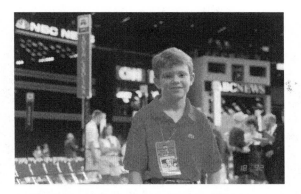

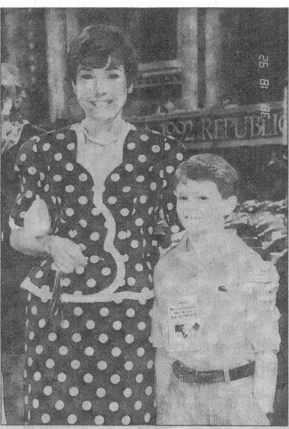

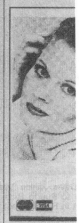

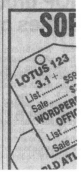

At the convention

Jake Driver, a 9-year-old resident of Spring Valley, stands with U.S. Trade Representative Carla Hills. Driver, who was one of the youngest volunteers at the Republican Convention held recently at the Astrodome, was a floor usher who showed delegates to their seats and checked floor credentials. Driver is a third-grade student at Saint Francis Episcopal Day School in Memorial.

Jake was recognized in the Houston Chronicle *as one of the youngest volunteers at the 1992 Republican National Convention.*

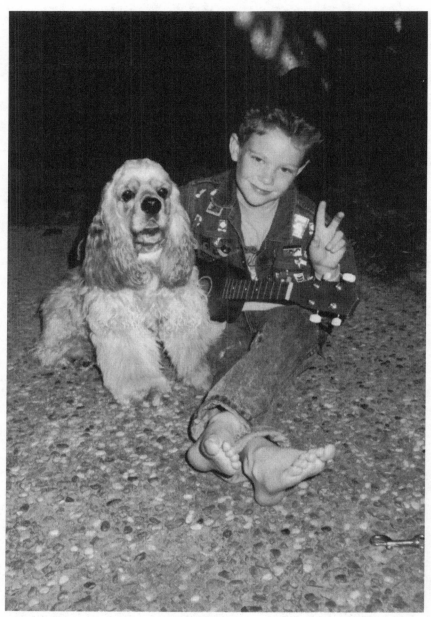

Jake's dog, Cutter, loved to hear him play his ukulele.

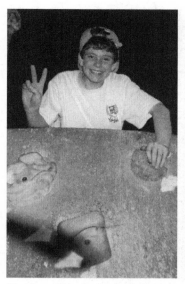

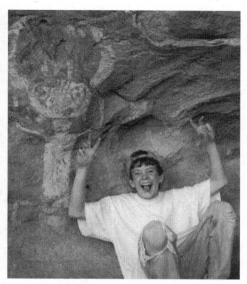

The physically and mentally challenging sport of rock climbing was a perfect outlet for Jake's boundless energy.

Jake flashes the victory sign after a successful climb at the Hueco Tanks in West Texas.

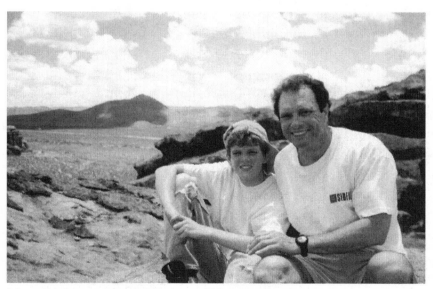

Jake and Mickey traveled to rock climbing and hiking sites throughout Texas.

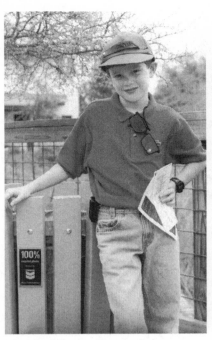

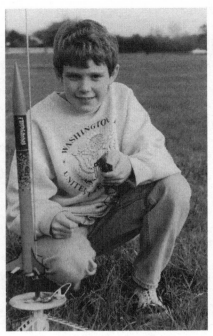

Jake helped clean up Houston during a
Chevron recycling drive.

Building and launching model rockets was a
great hobby during Jake's preteen years.

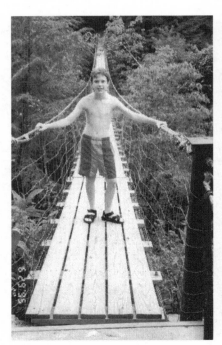

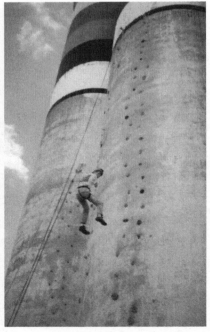

Jake crosses a suspension bridge at Falls Creek
State Park during a summer visit to Tennessee.

A grain silo in Dallas allowed Jake to hone his
rock climbing skills.

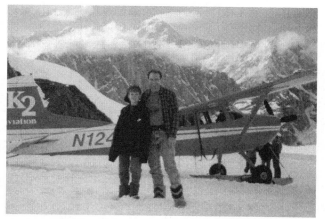

Landing on a glacier near Mt. Denali during a flightseeing tour was one of Jake's favorite memories of Alaska.

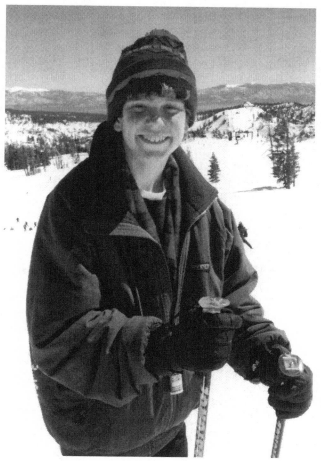

After his release from his first hospital stay, Jake and Mickey enjoyed a skiing weekend at Lake Tahoe.

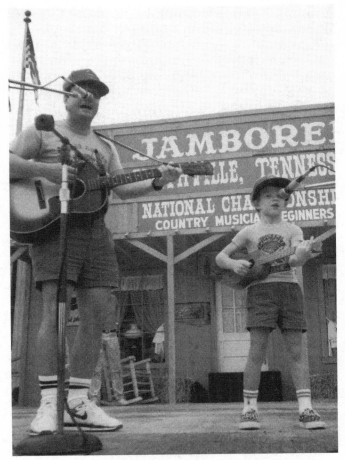

Jake's first musical performance was in 1988 when he sang Alabama's Song of the South *at the Smithville Fiddlers' Jamboree.*

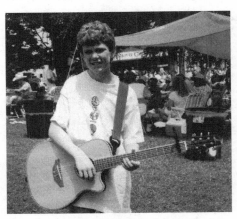

Jake returned to the Smithville Jamboree many times after his first appearance, always bringing his guitar.

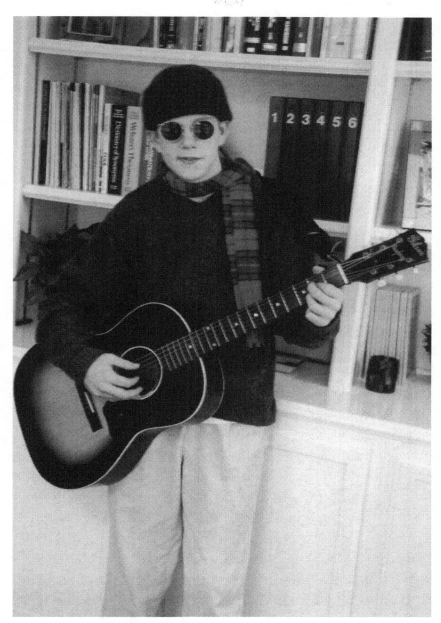

Jake plays the same guitar his grandfather, Bo Driver, played on the Grand Ole Opry.

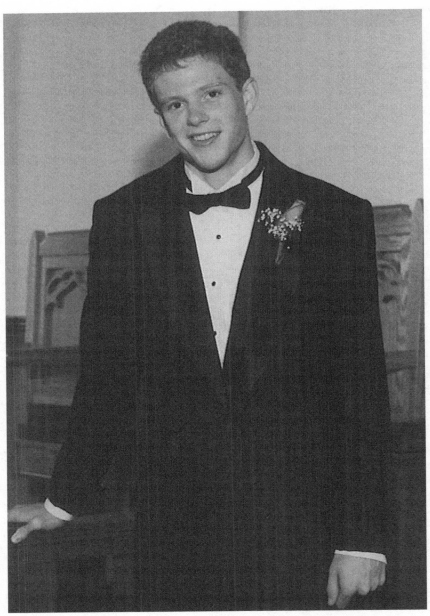
Jake served as the best man in Mickey and Debbie's nuptials on July 1, 2000.

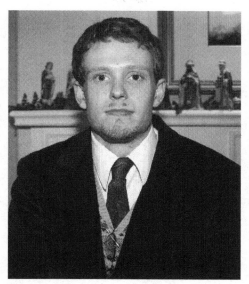

Jake turned up in his best attire for a Christmas party at the home of Jim and Mary Boyles.

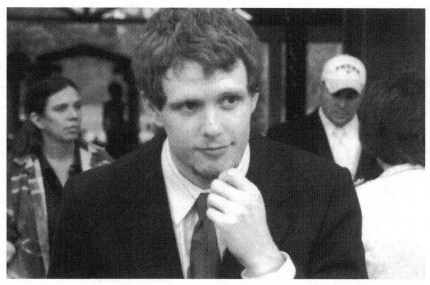

Jake was clean-shaven most of the time, but he also experimented with mustaches and goatees.

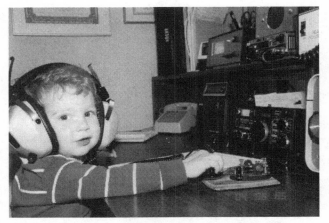

Even at age two, Jake could tap out his name in Morse Code.

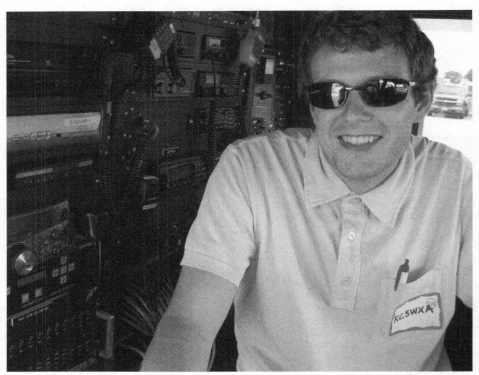

As his problems intensified, Jake's love of amateur radio seemed to grow. This photo was taken during the Texas City Hamfest in 2007 when Jake toured the American Red Cross Emergency Communications van.

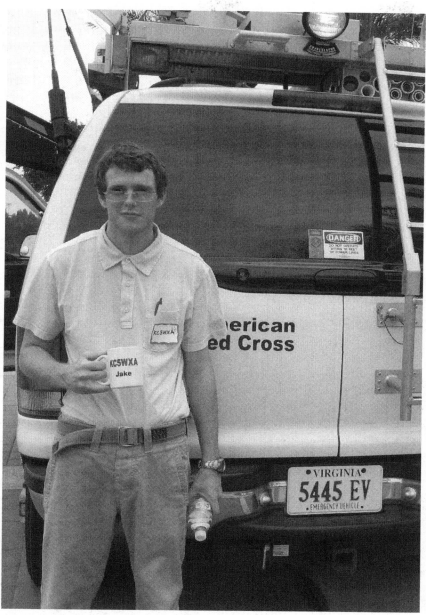

Jake was proud of his new coffee mug with his call sign, KC5WXA, on it. Jake attended the Texas City amateur radio "Hamfest" in 2007.

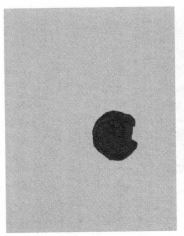

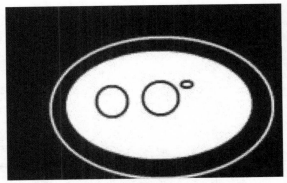

Jake called this piece of digital art "God's self-portrait."

Jake's oil painting "The eye of God"
was completed in January 2008.

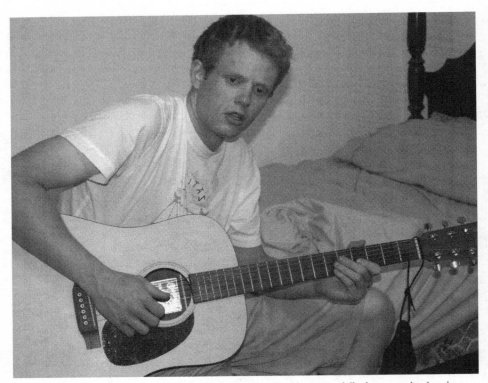

Over time, Jake became an accomplished guitarist. As he refined his guitar skills, his music developed
a raw bluesy sound.

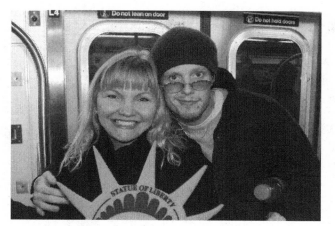

Debbie and Jake rode the New York subway after a long day of sightseeing and shopping during the Christmas holidays 2006.

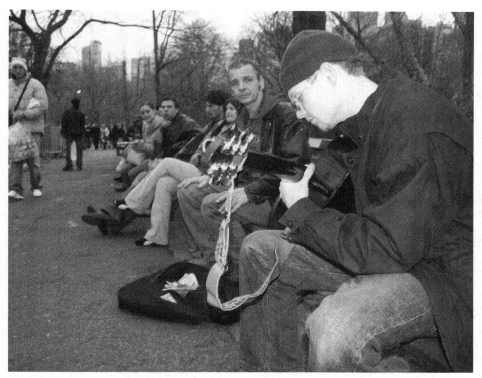

One of Jake's favorite moments was when he played several John Lennon songs at Strawberry Fields in New York's Central Park.

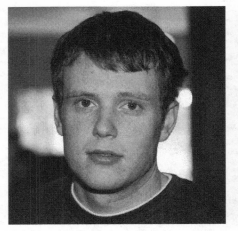
At Mommy Nell's house.

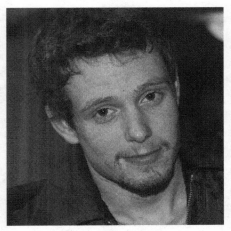
At the Opryland Hotel in Nashville.

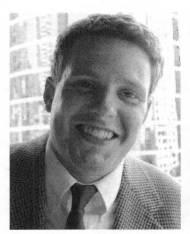
Dressed up after a court appearance.

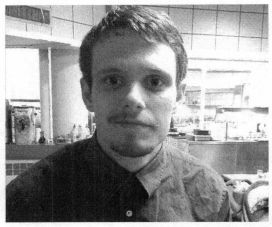
On the job at a Chinese restaurant in downtown Houston.

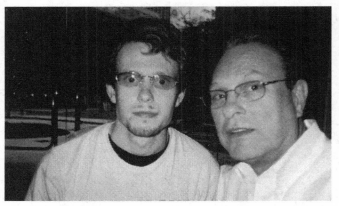
Jake visiting Mickey's downtown Houston office early in 2009.

the book of whispers

by
jake mcclain driver

POETRY TABLE OF CONTENTS

P i p e d r e a m   n o . 2

i saw perfect even circles divided by fives
the day the cumulus clouds came and
rectified my positions.

my soul removed

my worries feasting heartily

i spoke to them as though i knew,

but i didn't.

they drenched me with rainbow ice and cool crystal sorrows

gathering my jaded visions to move precious piercing tears

easing my heart

and washing with a vengeance
the lies I saw in the reflection of myself

it fell (it dropped)

the mirror opened up

and it occurred to me

<u>s w e e t   d r e a m s</u>

your kiss is worth a thousand deaths

please kill me again if it brings me one
length closer to your lips

even lying in my cold bed sleeping with
the window open to feel the icy chill upon
my breast

i crave a sea of blood

my own blood

I wish to bask in it with my flesh torn open
cascaded by flowing rose petals
and the smell of sexy sweat
teaming from the organs of young virgins

gathering at their parts

to ignite: their open seasons

       their wide flowers

A torn chest is distinguished
by the inscription of
innocence at the center

and in it lies your breath released
through your heart

come closer to me
i'll wash it all away

i grace the nape of your neck
allowing the gentle flow of sensation,
to follow the sweet sweep of our breath

all the way down

together we are tender

your smooth flesh, your face

are burning away at the intensity
of the moment

responding to my touch

we reach each other and turn inwards
creating a perfect cycle

<u>inspired in unison</u>

by a force of energy

found in a rhythm
we each share in our hearts

and when we return,

we will only be on the other side

there is no way out from here

but we don't mind...do we?

well i'm sorry

well i'm sorry
there was little i could do
moment came, i went down
fell right into you

got up to stand on my own two feet
but they had fallen asleep
my mind had too
fell right into you

ran up, ran down
ran on a straight street
took a drive, arrived alive
asked you for an address

you took a pencil from your bra

marked on the seat in my car

washed away a saturday,

and strangely took west to the movies

<u>b i r d s</u>

but it had little to do with the
birds' beaks locked in conjunction
with a corn nut.

(though they were lovers)

so i was not sorry to see them
devour it in unison,
knowing they would allow
the salt to dissolve in their beaks

to gather the juices together

they gather together

enough lather

to wash away all the markings
on the seat of my car with
birdpoop.

4

So I bring the girl into my closet where there
is only the carpet and a glass candle.

we sit across from each other and exchange meaningful

laughs and giggles   (dreambrushes of color)

because it's weird to be so private with another soul

the eyes do not bind the minds unless they are forced
to be naked and meet in agreement under contract

a pact,

that cannot be taken back (won't flip you no flap jack)

when we meet innocence's forgiven bunny rabbit (which is often mistaken
for a dirty habit)
bouncing through the forest (starkist)
we accidentally agreed to (torpedo)

swap a kinky saliva spit of tongues
unique to a chemistry
found only in the most holy of
laboratories

but we know nothing of each other's secret dimensions (not to mention)
and we know nothing of this which is why wonderful.

(so this stops, chop chop)

(chop chop)

we gaze (amaze)

eyes caught in the pale candlelight closet

in our hands (the two of us)

are chopsticks from our place (two of them)

and oatmeal boxes (two box, four chop)

we use them as drums. (I like the hums)

we sit there all night beating out rhythms (beat e a and a beat e a and a
beat e a ew ew yeha)

she sounds good cause, she's my girl
and she got grooves (and moves)

i can always dig her kind of crazy (even when i'm lazy)

she gives me this enticing glance (a chance for pants?)

like i should know what she's thinking

the beat goes on, i got you babe

never mind rewind
turpentine scent drag
it's a love rag
from Baghdad
unwind the twine
strawberry wine
finger dews dropping,
smooth clues
i could use,
perhaps confusion

what she really thinks is "i'm in love with you"

i am laid down
too involved
transfixed by her groove
and oblivious

she looks at me with the grace
of a fairy queen---light bouncing atop,

such soft edges

sexy there, too

constantly beating the drum,
giving herself to it,

making her actions a part of
rhythm which means
she got sweet love and sugar pumpkins
for her baby

and me just sitting there
kindly digging the cool way she does it

i'm gonna knock off my socks
kick back my cardboard conga
and bust out something sensationally
groovy over her rhythm

thinkin' "i love you"

it's perfect
and i beat my little sticks "groovy baby"

up and down
back and forth
in and out

she says " i love you too "

i'm hip to it

earache

there is a voice in the distance

all the more present now that i
have changed my state of mind

cool raindrops hit my window
one by one

and i count them all the way you
would count the heart pushes of females

i drown the way i have before

and the voice whispers in the distance

it rings clever notes that are my own,

but where did it live?

and why has it passed this way again?

it occurs to me that it is still in
the distances

in its own voice it whispers a revelation of its own
inside of time via me
inside of me via timeless
inside us all via the universe

but these curious moments
are the ones that drive it out

i like to listen,
so i listen

quietly,
for hours

2.

then of course comes you, we meet,
two universes collide,
as they must in the plot of every real story
that involves change

for a moment there is a still hanging
the breath is lost,
surely time has forsaken me

sorry now, "what did you say?"

<u>the fight</u>

all gentlemen are born secret warriors

sacred truths lay down swords at a round table
to preach civility

they agree to continue the fight on a safer field
exchanging armor for honor, dignity, and show
as one's own king

fine laden minds tip their hats to blood
only to please their mothers
who taught them well

of course, even the chemistry of these devices
has allowed soullessness to dilute the concentration
of purpose

media rain now withers the roof of the house

the tools have become so misrepresented
and the fight so large

that the words have developed the (roughened)
sharp jagged edges of ancient weapons

i used to be valiant as a knight,
i carried a sword avenging
the righteousness of the kingdom

now, peaceful as my princes sorrow

i carry a guitar and my words
avenging the innocence of my heart
and that which makes anyone laugh or cry

join me those who wish to stand upon the mountain,
and show your face to god

join me now

join the brotherhood

<u>d e e p e n</u>

how many words in the current language are like "grace"

are like "sweet"

are like "angel"

there is only one word for "love" in any language

and only one definition for "grace" in the dictionary

perhaps we're all saying the same thing

perhaps not

we're only human

do we mean what we say?

do we feel what we mean?

is there a rhythm to that?

words are hard to kill

in fact, words will never die

people will die

rocks will not die

they will wither

the pages will wither

you make hammers out of rocks

hammers are tools

words are mind hammers, thought nails

if i really didn't like you i might hit you on the head with a hammer

for lack of a better tool to deepen the blow

if i could blow you away,

that would solve this whole hammer equation with one easy touch
$1 + 1 = 1$

(together you have three:

the truth, you and me)

Earth

when my soul falls in,
it's as though i fall down

i'm connected to the ground

cool sweet earth in me, (like the trunk of a tree)

i like to open up, i like to get closed down

a very satisfactory bubble surrounds the sound around

      aura flora, deep tea

i am the ocean, and the ocean is me

unplug the stoppers and sink deep, there's nothing here you can keep

let it seep sea sap, I'll just sit and nap

<u>h a n g i n g   o n   m a r i l y n</u>

it's that moment where you inhale,

do it easily from beginning to end,
let it pass to the next note,

and know nothing of your actions,

or you have failed.

marilyn's lips radiate urgent emergency energies
from the beginning of time

star gazing pure light obsesses her body

she is the "original" woman

she is the desire of my manhood
and my blood

those who giggle,
those who entice me,

those who giggle enticingly

(it's all really somephtin')

i borrowed her pink plastic glasses

full at heart and pure are this breed of goddesses

              she stands in the kitchen

America's sweet teenager has grown to be my wife

passion priestess burning goddess
sun glaze fire blazing bright spark
torching my intricate insanity

after twenty years, the dragon lady is still jealous

even if i carried the spirit of nobility
she would leave me breathless

indeed she has left me breathless.

      it's odd when there are no separations

her love is the "original" love

i am the chosen one

she points a picker flashing my sign

an outstretched gloved lady finger
lends its perfection to my position

instantly i am obsessed

could it be so quick?

i am hung well

      i am hanging

she beckons, her breasts are beacons

i would never be so foolish as to tell myself i'm in control

i'm drawn in hanging

instant eternity
savvy solitude
sweet sex

and i fall all over her again,
i fall all over marilyn.

Kodak

i take a toke and poke out a poem

perfect pictures,

       built on faint memories

like the birdcage i dreamed

(It's more than a birdcage, of course)

it's an entire universe
as describable as a color

red is red

dream is birdcage

<u>w h i s p e r s</u>

it's funny, i've completely left my body

(those who really know me will understand best, of course)

right now you're seeing me "relatively well"

some secret part of you sees my secret part of me

some secret part of you is being pissy, pissed off at me

your energy undertow is pissing in my direction

it's funny,

if i were a baby, freshly fallen to the ground

i'd be crying right now

and on some secret dimension

where i was born and where i will die

I'm crying sweet, innocent, precious, baby tears

right now,
my mind is only comforted by the sound of myself
crying in the background

crying in heaven

giving me the energy to keep talking and walking along

i'm very good at being relatively well

time will change your body,
time does little to change your heart

unless you learn to open and let yourself in,
the way you opened and let them in.

but sometimes it's hard out there,

sometimes it's cold

sometimes it seems easier to speak
to strangers about souls

so they won't know about "true you"

what your mind's rushing through
which dream are we on?

oh yes, of course

the red one

with an intangible tinge of white light,

that was where i was that night.

<u>n i p p l e s</u>

so....anyway, this blond girl waltzes about here
dreamily moving about

the moveable intricacies of a changing reality
day by day

i've known her before
the way the lights atop her head
attach themselves to whatever beams brightest (for the moment)

always focusing on two or three big points, kept secret

forcing energy into the whole (often beautiful)

i've known her in a past life, we grew up together

and she knows me

so whenever we meet in space and time,

the reaction is always the same

i grab her breasts and begin to massage her nipples

pretending she's an etch-a-sketch

my conciseness becomes a scrolling dot,

drawing lines on her mind in the spirit of the past

it seems (as always) the memories have changed

but the little residue remains so the energies can be retraced and thusly, we met

we talked over coffee.

A: "you know a long time ago meeting people you hadn't
    viewed in a long time used to be a totally
    different experience"

B: "really? that sucks"

the thing about poetry is it's just there

in the air

who initially inhaled the essence of the truth's breath,
and was deemed trustworthy by the grace behind its rhythm?

was it you or was it me?

well we'll just have to see

i promise, times a plenty

and there can be no secrets in heaven

<u>r e m o t e   c o n t r o l</u>

i've lined up 564 commercial free perspectives,

and if i don't like the station,
i just change the channel

my mood ring changes color
from black and white to green

i have the desire to lift the cup

i withdraw the remote and signal

the infrared beam bounces through
the cups glass spectrum

shattering the cup in frequency
five – two – three

but lifting it to frequency five- two- four

which is my current destination location place

amazing marvels these remote control elevators

<u>g o d</u>

i see the wind

as it brushes through the trees

rustling the branches, the leaves

swooping down to sweep up the fallen pine needles
and carry them away

i see the wind

the wind is beautiful

the wind is like god

<u>b l u e s m o k e</u>

the musical experiment had gone array

and concluded in vast expansive explosions.

colorbombs graced the consciousness

for a fortnight.

bring a brainquilt,

knit it carefully

with inexpensive thread.

the golden needle does tire (still leaves its wire)

fine thin twine (wine)

drunk together on the astral plain

they attained real rain,

in their membranes forever

girl i won't mention

the grasp of us from behind the wildfire,

the madness in my being,

the outlet of my soul,
the outlet of my soul,
the outlet of my soul,

babe i can just pour it all over you,

tastes like honey

i like to breathe your warm breath
inches from your face,
cold as ice, near the frozen ocean

we are on the blanket alone,
in the most comfortable of distances,

crystal clear

star shine, sweet wine
i lost mine, in you

now you know

I am fearful, I am very very fearful of what i will do next

I have an open flesh wound,

I'm in a white room,

with a tiny cross the size of a plus sign.

it smells like antiseptic and me

seems i have placed little effort into eternity

i must contemplate it quickly

so many places to start, all of them frightening

the tunnel has opened, you will be judged upon the impulsiveness of your
thoughts

by the universe (with feet and a face if you wish)

you think you will sleep for a long time

instinctively,
do you do up or down?
happy or sad?
peace or confusion?

down, and the tunnel returns you to a whole new earth

up, and you beat out all the scanable waves of the spectrum

Gaze intently, he cometh with nature
and each vision shall see
and they which raised with vengeance
against the makers of the rains
and all the earth's mighty wonders.
He who hath risen,
in perfect harmony with one and other,
shall wail because of love in its mighty wrath
ever so,
Amen

true confessions of the
breakfast baboon

clean tangerine, marmalade mixture

open buttery crust pouring heavy wisps
into the crunchy chew

i enjoy the forest

i enjoy the wild sweet nectar
of free growing sporadic fruit

I get off foraging like Tarzan

i like the air in between
the cheetah cloth covering my loins

i especially enjoy beating my chest
and making that Tarzan noise

i'm going to pull a comic book clark kent

human nature by day

monkey nature by night

Superhero Forest Forager in Tarzan uniform

i leave in the early hours of dawn
by swinging from the vine
off the ledge of my apartment building

i arrive on time for my appointment with
the possums, squirrels, raccoons, and wise owls

the birds consume the space between
the branches of the trees
which appear green with leafy light
(via a "natural" glow)

we are ready – run! gather!

take from the forest in the night!

return the ecological cycles!

the wild gifts shine bright lights, (don't take the bad fruits)

their scents consume my senses, no worry

i am sensual, i do my duty with love

i remove the loin cloth
and close the filled ziploc sacks

i could live forever this way

i say we tear down the buildings,
            and the structure,
                    and all the obvious paved roads that imprison the
                    indestructible dirt

i say we teach this in school

Foraging 101

but who am i to say anything?

i'm just a guy dressed like tarzan
who likes to forage

(that's what school has taught me)

if you need me again you know what to do, (beat your chest and yodel)

and from now on,
when you see me in my loincloth,

just call me Tarzan

not monkey boy

i hate it when you call me monkey boy

hang loose blue caboose

i've got a blue caboose.

i say there's no use in it.

why's it hang loose?

dreamcicle icecrystals
and immaculate sex

and, though always lost in heaven,

i must ask:

where would i be without my blood?

where would i be without the magic healing
powers of mother nature?

i'd be a scab with no body

would crave no existence

defiant is death, and impossible

wander wayfarer

and continue aimlessly

like you walk about

aimlessly

like nighttime bathroom breaks on camping trips (alone)

just pissing in the wind

piss a happy wind please

<u>t h e   s c e n e</u>

everything is groovy – like a movie

you are allowed to float along with a senseful flow

in how many instances aside from your own? (none)

every man woman and child
indexed by tab dividers of your own design

and referred to, by you

accordingly,

inside your mind

inside your universe

<u>r e f l e c t i o n s</u>

i hear only the voices inside my head
and am otherwise, alone

i am delirious

i am not at the helm

who is the captain of this ship?

i am a madman, i am crazed

i am furious at boundaries

my hair crawls with weevils,

it expands in sharp dirty wisps

it covers all the red markings on my skin

it is dangerous

it extends an invitation

it sparkles insanity

how long have i been wild eyed?

how long have mirrors really fascinated me?

i cannot die, it is impossible

i can do anything i want

i'm not even the owner of this vessel

penelope is an angel

she drifts through my window on saturdays
to help me rearrange my ambitions

she reminds me of women
and gives me a couple of girls
to toy with for a while

they are lovely creatures

she refills my empty sack and cleans my room

she cooks a good meal
she does the laundry
she vacuums

she disappears and comes again on saturday

i love that smell

but exchanging it for the smell of sexy breath

and semen, returns it to the demons

took it out did you? i saw your urge

they were dancing naked in the forest

there is no real storybook innocence here on earth

would you care to go down with me?

we could laugh at the fools together,

while waiting for opportunities to produce the smell

make it love and share a universe, if not

it's been fun. (really)

were joining the dancers and dancing
along the lines of a magnificent figure eight

it will not end until either you or i fall down

but we knew we'd be separated
by either
ourselves or death one day

so it should come as no surprise

trip to the brief whimsical extreme

i don't care if there's a dog barking in there.

i'm going in just like the rest of them,

i will forfeit nothing,

we'll all burn in hell together

such is my vengeance.

you are perverted preachers, selfish servants, torturers, executioners,

devils, villains, fiends, you are horrid creatures of the darkness

you are ugly monsters,

i will drink your blood and purify my desires

i will piss you out

and i will flush you away

you will think you have me,

i will let you think you have me

and i will return you

i will throw your shit and fuck you up

wicked beast, you will fall back into the putrid pile from which you came

you'll burn in your guilty rancid stench

you will be frightened by the word forever ...

don't torture yourself with thoughts of being saved,

i have forgotten you exist all together

<u>Kum-by-ya</u>

when you truly have no words because
you're trying to describe a color

plain as damn day

when you want to hit them
with your heart

when you are constantly pursued by nagging angels

you'll know then,

i'll be right there waiting for you,

come, join me,

you are the chosen one

one for guys like you
(you know who you are)

the stewpot has been heating quite some time,

it's boiling now

the steam is thick,

billows,

white puffs, ozone

the spheres atmosphere blazes in heat

and the virgin takes the blue pill for the first time

she has grown,
now she will beg us to attend to her needs

she has swallowed her cycle

empowered, it will divide her mad unless she channels it

i have recently become a member of the republican soccer mom's
agenda aggression passion depravation prevention society

we have a simple motto: make love to them now
shock their edges
keep her glowing
surprise is safety

to the gang of wicked men who walk this world without emotions,
to those who set out to create their own world
with a perception of their own presumption,

doesn't the world just seem to unravel to you,........ it's all money

<u>r e v e r b e r a t i o n</u>

i know of no innocence greater than love,

i know of no time quicker than purity.

if i was completely deaf i would live alone inside my mind

and i would feel your presence

you would walk into the room and i would sense your anger

their voices have disturbed you again, fool

you have only yourself to be angry at,

the thoughts are your own

m y m y

i see that you have been sitting in the sun,

it has ripened the cherries in the middle
of the soft part of your round muffins

you are a very pretty creature

i like all your extremities

you must feel very good

i'd like to make you feel very good

i retain all the qualities of smooth silky butter (i'm on a roll)

i have been churning for some time now

i am ready

i am like butter

i would like to bath you,
to baste you rather

the sun has baked your buns

i will butter them!

you little lady name shall be muffins,

i've come to milk your honey butter creamers, miss muffins

teacher said it was a poem

this light's too bright

i like my night light

it turns on automatically, it has a little sensor

it's cute, i like my night light

<u>getting dressed</u>

i would like to try out my new coat
on the sensual visuals,
of the creatures from this new day

i have begun to shed my snake skin scales in rapid cycles

perpetual regenerating

touch me,

i will start to grow you.

looking too sharply

i have arrived on time and there are no dreams left

kiss me before the moment is over and i cannot (to end it here)

i have a second chance, i thank eternity

the sharpening

quick, i have become clever

sleep never, be awake forever

i am all that i can fathom,
i count the moments in timed triplets

careful celerity, cold cucumber

the phone rings before i dial your number

touch me soon and at your own risk

if you don't,

it's your loss

3

a kiss is the sign of an open lingering

if it's invited, it's often very clean and fresh

like produce, like lettuce

it's like, i like the lock a lot,

sucking the flaps

enclosed in the caves

the breath mixture like the relationship
between two warm perky volcanoes
and the warmth of steam
in the sky's clouds above you

it is only appropriate to close your eyes,

and fly into her

seems stupid to say

the sun bounces up and down
the blue coastal waters
like a fun red ball

of course: sun
            waters

there must also be infiniti

old farts

i try not to listen to the jaded perceptions
of life presented to me by old farts

best i can do is charm them

let them bask in my presence for a bit

i have no fear for them

i just sit and wait for their cheeks to
turn in magnificent awestruck wonder
at it all

and when they're little old crumply people

sitting together on a comfy sofa

napping in peace

snuggled cozily under a warm blanket

with their little noses poking through

having sweet dreams of the marvelous
quality of the air conditioning

and the ten thousand some odd channels
they'd lost count of long ago

they'll awake to find us, greeting them politely
with smiling faces and cookies

and they'll have a good marvel
at the kindness of our generation

because it's love

and we throw it around a lot
and sometimes we stumble

but it's more fun that way

the last whisper

and when your hungry son is done

and mass confusion has begun

you'll know it's true,

i was the one

and know i'm through

now i'm just a little voice in you

day is done,

but still not overcome

<u>n i g h t   f l i g h t</u>

a natural bird flew over my head

i plucked it from the sky

i took its spirit in my godly hand

i shot it with word arrows,
piercing its heart with my
peaceful poetic vibrations

i have died before and will die again

in between and during it all

i merely exist and become born

our souls exchange the color blue
as brothers in righteousness

the unity of creation

we are bound (and bonded) in spirit

i will not kill you,
yet you will be killed

i will merely gesture
toward the dropping hammer
of mortality

you bird, need not thoughts so complex as these

you will fly, just fly

you will be oblivious in oblivion

i have implanted the spirit of peace in you,
            the spirit of awakening in you,

you will pass far into the night

you shall strive to become eternal here on earth,
as an image in its heart

i have struck the disc now

it radiates the energies you shall
carry upon your journey

it reunites you with your godliness
and your body

you know only, only knowing, at all

i have entrusted you with the spirit of peace, bird,
i have entrusted you with the spirit of peace, bird,

fly to each of the reaches of this earth

fly to the dark corners of time

illuminate them!

fill us till we are filled and we are full

and you are emptied

you will die bird,

but you shall live whole,

in all of us

<u>thought</u>

i think that, what i think is that,
i think, i am thinking. (don't cha think so)

in the end

when everybody's dancing

the dance is free

we'll keep the secret
just you and me

won't let them know it's our fault

what do you say old pal?

<u>o n e   f o r   t h e   J u n g i a n</u>

indeed all things are present,

you are whole

but be forewarned

the thoughts you elaborate upon in action

are the doors your soul dwells upon in spirit

so be forewarned

that conversation is an action

and you live a life,

you live a life that entails more than watching

god does not care about your notes,

he already knows what you wrote,

and so do i

i've been watching too

all i'm really asking you to do,

is accept your dreams for what they are

<u>these media eyes</u>

all my time for you,
is just scissors and glue

rip open, cut through gashes in my heart

grasp my whisper
pull me apart, run me through
leave me, depart

run run run
but it's circles you see
i'm runnin' through you,
your runnin' through me

and so together we shall dream,
like two potatoes watchin' the same screen
(it's more congenial than it may seem)

kind for a day

i grew to know there were friends,
who were my brothers

and ladies who were my lovers,

i became a kind king that day

<u>n i b b l e s</u>

i like little snack packages,
convenient cookies

when i get the nibbles

i'll nibble on you

i like little ladies
gracious loves easy progress

i get the munchies,
and i'm hungry

i like to eat till i'm full,
and i'm bottomless

<u>t h i s m o r n i n g ' s h i g h</u>

there is at present, no past

it's a junkies comfort zone

yesterday is only a concept

time exists only here on earth,
and i rarely exist there with it

i've got "original energy"

i am god

there are no memories

only beginnings, with the convenience of words

i am jumping constantly and could never
interrupt the action to question the pedestal
from which i sprang

and that's good, like in heaven, with angels

i am whole and new

and that's really good

<u>true confessions of the dream king</u>

it was open the day you left

like in the wind, it carries easy

move to tracing, follow

early woolen pollen balls

clothed eternity

fields of grass,
fields of grass,

satisfying human sweat
basks underneath the sun
you'll never know while sleeping

i smoke a cigarette and drink a cup of coffee

for lack of a phone call

the phone's no longer you

it's them

they want to move me along
-on to a new daydream

why?

two days, seven years,
seems no difference

what's the change?

haven't i always been here?

and now i'm here without you

it's that much colder

like the urgency behind the blue pills
exposing the flipside

<u>f l i p s i d e</u>

this moment's all too satisfying

you are now unlimited

like the goddess who enchanted me
with an early glance on the first occasion

you allow my mind to multiply

i flow madly, passionately wild

i could become addicted to coffee
i could become addicted to the wind

rarely are the moments so sweet

rarely is my window so open

everything sends in seasons

i shall see you, when you have gone

i shall see you when you have come again

logical balloons

you bought me a big red balloon

i left it in my room

it got winded and pooped out (whizzed away)

it lied, cold, dead, defeated, and shriveled on the floor

if our love had faded all this inevitable dying would mean terrible omens,

now it's cute (because it pooped out)

the world is a breeding ground for love and death

but you're stupid if that reflects your depth

my soul outwits my mind 24/7

<u>calling her</u>

now begin the procedure,
now procure,

now turn around and shut the door,

do me, do me, do me

like you've never done before

i need more
i want more
give me more

more girl more
more girl more
more girl more

tuck and roll

a little thing happened to me today
that i wasn't quite able to process

so i tucked it away

like a nick nack in a pocket

i'll find it later,

like a nifty nick nack in a pocket

i suppose i secretly enjoy surprising myself

it's neat,

(it's an even grove, like a cool key,
            peachy king
            round ripe bright like
a hunky dory sugared cherry
and so much other with
sugar on top)

<u>fertile insanity</u>

a. so you got the bastard in the jail cell,
   in the restraining jacket

you got him under control

you're very impressive and powerful

go ahead, let me see you make him think

why isn't he thinking

make him think dammit

b. so the time had come,
   and they finally arrived
and they had decided to kill me

they asked me to say a few words

i said "i've had beautiful dreams"

9

it is the inevitable hour and the mad men will do it again

i've been staying in, trying to think without using words

it's great

once you practice

practice makes perfect

perfect practice makes perfect sense

there go the madmen again

arguing analytics

always arguing analytics

<u>s t o p</u>

comfortably alone

wallowing through pillows of my own

to smash into my own self ordained barriers face first

and lie, defeated

in my own pillows, without motion for minutes

and i recharge this easy fall

by staring at these walls

still smokin'

they could only stop the flood
by burning bountiful bills

to see the difference in the colors they make,

while beautifully ablaze

the corded love burns with you and above you, as you
(have you found it yet?)

the loose one hangs heavy (obviously),
always extinguished in the end

later date

(1A)
you're taking the soul drug?

ignite the night with intoxication
and hail it properly, as an American

(2B)
so i fly today....   yeha i flew ..... it was great

the sky, was it high?

fuckin monstrous say i

a big big sky?
was it all you had ever hoped?

oh no – for that would have killed it

you see, hope is like a starfish

satisfaction is the ocean
energy is oxygen

can't ever balance everything out huh?

it gets easier, as you discover oxygen

and everything that breathes,
has its own way of breathing

because life is arbitrary

so you got high?

just call me the rocket baby!

there's two of us here if i'm not mistaken
no there's three: you just showed up (4)
(oh yes, were thoughts not people) (5)
that's four, four fucking thoughts (6)
no that's five (7) ...wait .. (8)
don't you see we just keep growing? (9)

so you got high?
yeha man i got high

 shut up you two, i'm tryin to sleep

i'm sleeping only on intense dimensions

the forest

you do what you do,
always doing, you are you

when the water is still you may
see your reflection

the juggle thinks little of the objects
though there are three: (body, mind, soul)

float upon the water, walk a-cross it

and you will recognize and bond with
spirits who stay afloat

the water will shine

inside and outside
in the world
out of the world
you are one among many

but the light and life
illuminate those whose
faces are awakened,
with radiant purity

amidst it all,

shine in you, you will shine
inside and outside, with smiles

2

you are everything

can't take me away
can't take me away
but cha do

and i am you

twists these lips to curls for
you girl

completely do
complete with you
you complete me

<u>awning daytime coffee buzz</u>

though i sit cross-legged in the nice light of an upside down noon moon,

my hands proceed to make swim-like motions
in this present daytime distress
of feeling the thoughts slip from my brain
as though they were being wrung through a tightly clinched fist
and chased by a man i didn't like
the way my eye chases the remainder of a light bulb

twinkle trip

<u>A</u>

i suppose i secretly enjoy running though a maze of mirrors when
nobody's lookin'

if i come about a bomb, and it bombards me......it blows

straight shooting up like comet trails in the ice

blast balloon where no mirror can hide its reflection

so the maze is consumed with light

<u>B</u>

i am numb today

though not fully

because the sheets are not covering my head
the way this light is

i furiously figuratively pound upon my brain to keep from being lost
inside it

i'm searching for something, the words are tedious

(fuck i'm between worlds again)

{just passing says hello: when i was three and i threw up (random)}

and so snickey winky inky ding dong (i look up) (that guy's gablabering
and he knows it)

{come to stay says: lying in those arms}

(the bomb blows up and the mirrors are consumed)

come to stay says: snickey winky inky ding dong (but i don't care, it
makes perfect sense)

i'll be like this for an hour or so

my blue eyed son

1
i have chased my blue-eyed son to the foothills
he ran fast and far ahead of me

my spirit followed him to the joy of his play

i knew the foothills would be exciting

i prepared a cushion of laughter
he heard the angel's voices as he
smiled and followed them

and he learned of his existence in this lifetime

2
i have chased my blue-eyed son to the mountains
he cursed me and begged me to let him go alone, (he's so brave)

my spirit followed him to the peace of his meditations

i knew the mountains would be cold

i prepared a cushion of truth
he sat high upon it, he sat righteous

and he learned to be pure in this lifetime

3
i have chased my blue-eyed son to the sun.
he told himself he went alone

yet my spirit followed him to the reality of his dance

his fair skin bathed in the warm sunlight as it became dark with the
prolonged intensity of exposure

i prepared a cushion of beauty and he danced upon it in grace

and he learned to feed himself in this lifetime

<u>4</u>
i have chased my blue-eyed son to the end.
there he could not deny my presence

i awaited the finished product

he came to me perfectly
the way i had dreamed he would

he said "mother's love"

i was broken, released, whole again

and then, no longer needed to chase him

while he politely came to visit.

<u>5</u>
one world, all souls equal in the end

even mothers

even sons

all is one

<u>a true poet speaks</u>

if you'd like to revere me, (or a potato for that matter)

revere love,
      spirit
      soul
      unity
      brotherhood
      creation
      god

i just like doin' it i could do it all night

just for the natural rush

i can take as much credit for my creations
as my parents can for my flesh and blood

Romans 12:2

And be not conformed to this world;
but be ye transformed by the renewing of
your mind, that ye may prove what *is* that good,
and acceptable and perfect will of god.

<u>s u d d e n l y</u>

when it comes suddenly it comes with grace

i understand that it is raining and nothing more

i gave up science long ago but that has little to do with anything now
(it doesn't take long to become awestruck by the stars)

i'd like to marry you

i need that in order to keep myself sane

and we've got to stop meeting like this

because it occurs to me lately that my entire consciousness
can become a product of a little clock i keep inside
that measures time in terms of our togethers

this constant ticking is driving me crazy

it's been there all these lengths
like the chemistry in each lover's original glance

you cannot duplicate that feeling

and you are the purple velvet sky

fate will draw us closer, i pray

for the clouds are lovely,
but i prefer the suns

car wash

interscope freeway transfer
tripping daisy's red rain scarlet velvet cushion
and the open wides

you eat all you can bite off (it's soft)

purple ocean princess peacetube
like the one you had yesterday

born bravely an hour ago,
 heart in hand
wandering far and deep

keeping only dreams it seems odd

whisper rushes, a cloudy days velvet vapors

hissing to the countless waves of the rainbow comfort pulse

partially ignited by the princes' sorrowful princess dreams

partially flamed by you, here, in the now

vulnerable by the light

one for the window

one for the door

i'm one for the girl, and no one more

<u>to taste the day</u>

i broke a new egg
in the early morning
on a clean plate's edge
which reflected the
awning glory of the
sun's opening beams.

it was fresh and crisp, slicing

like a lime

and sourpuss' tangy lemon morning cocktail

the memory of atoms passing along my tongue

to my tasters, my tasty taste buds

i taste that same bitter sweetness

this day shall be savory indeed.

<u>m e n o m o r e</u>

i release my wicked smile, i no longer need an ego grin

i smile upon you, i smile in wholesome heaven

take these astral glasses: steal them from yourself, and give them to you

i have contracted warmth

darkness does not exist, though it does

one has to do, to do not

light shines in my space

i have filled my bubble with the warmth
of me and all my angels

one cord connects me, both: to earth and heaven

you could only be jealous of me,
because i have more of you than you do

but who are you but the universe?

and who am i but the universe?

i think we are all light beings

i am light

and anything that exists, exists upon the spectrum

the real world is nothing more than a mental television
receiving a broadcast from the dreamworld

matter is a slow manifestation of light,
the creative process in this dimension is tedious:

dream then build, dream then build

those who follow the awakened seek
the speed of creation that exists in the dreamworld

so they may fix the earth, it needs to breathe

radio waves bend and groove at the command of your voice

your eyes vibrate your soul

you send you anger, i see your anger
the vibration exists

you send you love, i see you love
the vibration multiples

to cast

i shall cast the wind upwards,
        casting upwards into the wind

i shall cast off a fine flying kite

i shall cast a spell

the wind is open for casting

i forecast fortunate fishing

i shall cast into the ocean

i'll hear the angels say "cast away!"

i wish to feel peace beneath the flow

and then to cast

i wish for more wishes,
        so i can catch more fishes

it's better to teach a man to fish,

than to fish for free

sounds fishy to me

fish from the sea are always free

a world to cast into,

a soul to return you

the distances

break open an eggshell universe

engage the spaces

forget babylon

employ the beyond

tear away all the walls,
in the hallways,
in the sky

say "i am one" three times

begin to fly

let go lost ladies, look for the blind light

let away loss childhood dreamer

break open an eggshell universe

welcome to the distances

what you'll be saying to me now,
is what you'll be saying in the end

from here we are returned

begin again
born again
end again
die again
turn in

it's been a rough day

2786

the time has come,
        now buy me a dream

there's nothing more to say

i bought this world,

i bought a boat,

and now i'll sail away

meeting in conversation

it was a perfect example of citrus

a bright sunny orange

i have communicated an image of fruit,

from my mind to yours, on the astral plain

two universes meeting on
similar sectors of the same spectrum

exchanging frequencies

knowing the same frequencies were exchanged

a little like listening to music,

but more bourgeois and less precise
because there's a lot more to the universe
than just fruit

because words are heavy tools.
buffers to soulful lightning

and this is how we talk

seems a lot of people should shut up

just hand me the orange

and say "i love you"

<u>o n e   f o r   t h e   d a r k n e s s</u>

shadows in the darkness,

impossible say i!

how have i these eyes,

to see me in the darkness
of this unholy night

my big bubble holds all the
secrets of the universe

i pray to the love between us,

and pray the hope will save us.

until then, i'll be content within my bubble
just hopping along,
hopping like a happy hippo

hopping a ground of dark water
which i can only hop above,

because i am not nothing,

i am love

the universe is all voices

yet it cannot speak for itself

it speaks through you

you are the universe

you seek the secrets of the universe

the way they seek you

you are the light,

the light is you

you are all beings

all beings are you

you know all the secrets of the universe

you know none of the secrets of the universe

though you as **one**, cannot be aware of both at <u>once</u>

you are the spirit of awareness

be aware of the highest point of awareness,
and all creatures shall desire to follow you

the spectrum is currently the most accessible
form of Infiniti

any expression of the soul must currently
be conveyed though heavy tools

all of which encompass *vibration*: the manipulation of the spectrum

talking, seeing, hearing, manipulating

conversation
music
dance
art
poetry

creation in this world is a product of the souls doing

expression of the soul is all that matters

we are moving upwards in awareness

always,

we may never go down, unless we forget
and make our souls isolated

awareness is infinite as the universe

the universe is infiniti

the universe is the universe

all is one

<u>piss on everything tomorrow's</u>
<u>saturday</u>

tiny authors

self-proclaimed prophets

poets, the lonely jewels

one step away from a pure death

walk this world with the wisdom a dying man

laugh at the fools becoming intoxicated

while we take for ourselves,
tiny guiltless pieces of heaven here on earth.

to see them all perfectly
to be them all perfectly

knowing very well you once
were them ......perfectly

for we have been all people,
and may speak for them

maintaining our poetic consciousness

knowing what lucky fools we are,

knowing our thoughts pass for poetry

<u>the distances continue</u>

knock, knock

whose there?

there's no in here but us scaredy rubber chickens
getting ready to cross the road
but having second thoughts because we're chicken

no now, really now

knock, knock

whose there?

there's no one in here

i no say no nothing

no, now really now

knock knock

whose there?

i could be anything,

but i could only be the universe

it's all ones and zeros from the bottom